FRACTURES OF THE
UPPER EXTREMITY

FRACTURES OF THE
UPPER EXTREMITY

EDITED BY

BRUCE H. ZIRAN

St. Elizabeth Health Center,
Northeastern Ohio Universities College of Medicine
Youngstown, Ohio, U.S.A.

WADE R. SMITH

Denver Health Medical Center
Denver, Colorado, U.S.A.

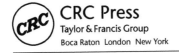

CRC Press
Taylor & Francis Group
Boca Raton London New York

CRC Press is an imprint of the
Taylor & Francis Group, an **informa** business

CRC Press
Taylor & Francis Group
6000 Broken Sound Parkway NW, Suite 300
Boca Raton, FL 33487-2742

First issued in paperback 2019

© 2004 by Taylor & Francis Group, LLC
CRC Press is an imprint of Taylor & Francis Group, an Informa business

No claim to original U.S. Government works

ISBN-13: 978-0-8247-4718-3 (hbk)
ISBN-13: 978-0-367-39484-4 (pbk)

Visit the Taylor & Francis Web site at
http://www.taylorandfrancis.com

and the CRC Press Web site at
http://www.crcpress.com

Preface

The region between the shoulder and wrist is an important part of the body, as without the upper extremity there is severe functional impairment. In many ways, such impairment is greater than the counterpart in the lower extremity; this is readily apparent by looking at the homunculus of the somato-motor regions of the brain. Realizing the societal impact of computers and the subsequent need for upper extremity use to operate such devices, one can easily imagine the impact on society. More and more people depend on and use the upper extremity for gainful and recreational purposes. The functional result of prostheses in the lower extremity is often better than that of reconstruction, but there are no equivalent products for the upper extremity. Thus, surgical reconstruction of the injured upper extremity is increasingly important—not only to patients but also to society.

Fractures of the Upper Extremity represents the culmination of outstanding work from our contributors. We have been fortunate to have some of the very best young surgeons and academicians contribute to this book. It includes chapters from both orthopedic traumatologists, who care for the majority of upper extremity injuries, and upper extremity surgeons, who focus exclusively on the upper extremity. Together, they have provided a nice spectrum of philosophies and approaches. We hope that this text will be useful to anyone involved in the care of the upper extremity, from the student to the therapist, and from the general practitioner to the cutting-edge surgeon. We would like to thank and acknowledge the numerous people who helped us organize and complete this arduous task. We also thank our teachers and mentors, who have taught us so much and allowed us to do what we do.

Bruce H. Ziran
Wade R. Smith

Contents

Contributors

Sam Akhavan, M.D. Department of Orthopaedics, Case Western Reserve University/University Hospitals of Cleveland, Cleveland, Ohio, U.S.A.

Mark E. Baratz, M.D. Division of Hand and Upper Extremity Surgery, Department of Orthopaedic Surgery, Allegheny General Hospital, Pittsburgh, Pennsylvania, U.S.A.

Rob Dawson, M.D. Division of Hand and Upper Extremity Surgery, Department of Orthopaedic Surgery, Allegheny General Hospital, Pittsburgh, Pennsylvania, U.S.A

Robert J. Goitz, M.D. Department of Orthopaedic Surgery, University of Pittsburgh Medical Center, Pittsburgh, Pennsylvania, U.S.A.

William Greer, M.D. Division of Hand and Upper Extremity Surgery, Department of Orthopaedic Surgery, Allegheny General Hospital, Pittsburgh, Pennsylvania, U.S.A

Brian M. Jurbala, M.D. Hand and Upper Extremity Surgery, University of Pittsburgh Medical Center, Pittsburgh, Pennsylvania, U.S.A.

Kirti Moholkar, M.S., F.R.S.C.I. Denver Health Medical Center, Denver, Colorado, U.S.A.

Carlos Mario Olarte, M.D. Department of Orthopedic Surgery, Hospital de San Jose, Fundación Universitaria de Ciencias de la Salud, Bogotá, Colombia

Greg M. Osgood, M.D. Department of Orthopaedic Surgery, New York Orthopaedic Hospital, Columbia-Presbyterian Medical Center, New York, New York, U.S.A.

Ian Pallister Denver Health Medical Center, Denver, Colorado, U.S.A.

Rodrigo Pesantez, M.D. Department of Orthopedic Surgery, Fundación Santa Fe de Bogotá, Universidad del Rosario, Bogotá, Colombia

Kevin J. Pugh, M.D. Division of Trauma, Department of Orthopaedics, The Ohio State University, Columbus, Ohio, U.S.A.

Melvin P. Rosenwasser, M.D. Department of Orthopaedic Surgery, New York Orthopaedic Hospital, Columbia-Presbyterian Medical Center, New York, New York, U.S.A.

Ioannis Sarris, M.D., Ph.D.* Department of Orthopaedic Surgery, University of Pittsburgh Medical Center, Pittsburgh, Pennsylvania, U.S.A.

Vishal Sarwahi, M.D. Department of Orthopaedic Surgery, New York Orthopaedic Hospital, Columbia-Presbyterian Medical Center, New York, New York, U.S.A.

John W. Shaffer, M.D. Department of Orthopaedics, Case Western Reserve University/University Hospitals of Cleveland, Cleveland, Ohio, U.S.A.

Wade R. Smith, M.D. Department of Orthopaedics, Denver Health Medical Center, Denver, Colorado, U.S.A.

Dean G. Sotereanos, M.D.† Department of Orthopaedic Surgery, University of Pittsburgh Medical Center, Pittsburgh, Pennsylvania, U.S.A.

Current affiliation: Department of Orthopaedic Surgery, Allegheny General Hospital, Pittsburgh, Pennsylvania, U.S.A.

†*Current affiliation*: Division of Hand and Upper Extremity Surgery, Department of Orthopaedic Surgery, Human Motion Center, Allegheny Orthopaedic Associates, Cranberry Township, Pennsylvania, U.S.A.

1

Dislocation and Ligament Injury of the Elbow and Forearm

Ioannis Sarris* and Dean G. Sotereanos†
University of Pittsburgh Medical Center, Pittsburgh, Pennsylvania, U.S.A.

The elbow is the second most commonly dislocated major joint, after the gleno-humeral joint (1). Recent biomechanical studies of the mechanism of injury in elbow dislocation as well as studies of elbow function have offered significant insight into the treatment of these injuries.

I. MECHANISM OF INJURY

Causes of elbow dislocation are (1) a fall on the outstretched hand, (2) a motor vehicle accident, (3) direct trauma, and (4) sports.

The mechanism of injury has been described as a fall on the outstretched hand with the shoulder in abduction. This produces an axial compressive force to the elbow because of the weight of the body. As the fall continues, the body rotates internally, forcing the forearm into external rotation (supination) and the elbow into valgus. The combination of these three forces (axial compression, supination moment, and valgus deformation) accurately explains the mechanism of posterolateral subluxation, which consequently leads to posterior dislocation (2) (Fig. 1).

The traditional description of the elbow dislocation mechanism—as being due to elbow hyperextension (3), with olecranon impingement causing a lever effect—inadequately explains the variations of the injury.

**Current affiliation*: Allegheny General Hospital, Pittsburgh, Pennsylvania, U.S.A.

†*Current affiliation*: Human Motton Center, Allegheny Orthopaedic Associates, Cranberry Township, Pennsylvania, U.S.A.

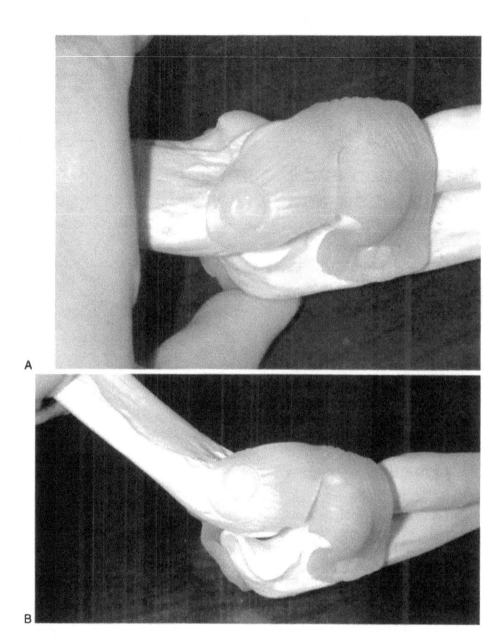

Figure 1   A to C. The combination of these three forces—axial compression, supination moment, and valgus deformation—accurately explains the mechanism of posterolateral subluxation, which consequently leads to posterior dislocation. D. Lateral radiograph of posterolateral dislocated elbow.

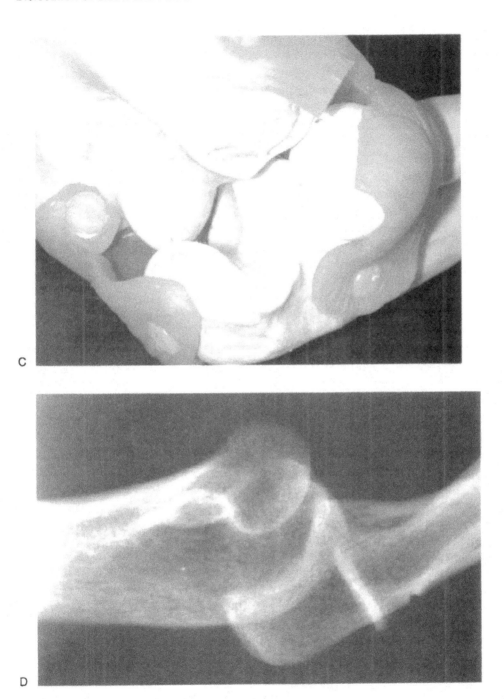

Figure 1 Continued.

The mechanism of injury for anterior dislocation is probably similar to that of posterior dislocation except for a forward rebounding response and excessive hyperextension. This allows the olecranon to unlock from the olecranon fossa or to be fractured and slide under the trochlea anteriorly.

Posterior elbow dislocation can also occur with the joint in flexion and requires a longitudinal axial load, resulting in radial head and coronoid process fractures. It was experimentally proven that posterior dislocation with the elbow in a semiflexed position could occur with combined valgus and external rotary stress, leading to medial and lateral ligamentous injury (4).

In children, the "pulled elbow" is a traction injury in which the head of the radius is pulled partially under the annular ligament while the forearm is pronated and the elbow is extended (5).

The mechanism of injury for divergent dislocation of the elbow involves high-energy trauma with disruption of the radiocapitellar, ulnotrochlear, and proximal radioulnar joints with rupture of the interosseous membrane, annular ligament, and joint capsule (6).

In elbow dislocations the soft tissue injury progresses in a circle-like pattern. First the lateral unlar collateral ligament is ruptured; afterwards the rest of the lateral ligamentous structures and the anterior capsule are torn; and then the medial posterior and ulnar medial collateral ligament rupture (2) (Fig. 2).

II. DIAGNOSIS

A. Classification

In children the term *pulled elbow* refers to the association between the radius and the annular ligament, an injury that is usually a result of joint hypermobility or ligamentous laxity. The entity of congenital radial head dislocation has also been described.

The main classification of acute elbow dislocations corresponds to the direction of the proximal radioulnar joint and olecranon displacement in relation to the distal humerus.

1. Posterior Dislocation

This is the most common type of elbow dislocation, where the proximal radioulnar joint dislocates posteriorly to the distal humerus. It can be medial or lateral, but this is irrelevant to the final treatment.

2. Anterior Dislocation

This is a very a very uncommon injury of the elbow, where the proximal radioulnar joint dislocates in front (anteriorly) of the distal humerus. It is usually seen in children (7), while in adults it is usually associated with an olecranon fracture.

3. Divergent Dislocation

This is a rare injury of the elbow, where the proximal radioulnar joint is disrupted with consequent rupture of the interosseous membrane, resulting in ante-

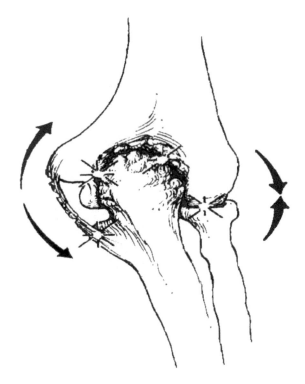

Figure 2   Circle-like pattern injury of the elbow dislocation. First the lateral unlar collateral ligament is ruptured; then the rest of the lateral ligamentous structures and the anterior capsule are torn; and finally the medial posterior and ulnar collateral ligament rupture.

rior dislocation of the radius and posterior dislocation of the olecranon in relation to the distal humerus. These injuries usually occur after high-energy trauma, but they can also be seen in cases of annular ligamentous insufficiency or in bony erosive conditions like rheumatoid arthritis (8).

Pure medial or lateral dislocations are likewise unusual.

Elbow dislocations can also be subdivided in to (1) simple dislocations without fracture and (2) complex ones with associated fractures. This subdivision is significant for the choice of treatment and for the prognosis of the final functional outcome.

B.   Associated Injuries

Associated injuries in elbow dislocations are very common (9–11). Fractures of the radial head and neck occur in 10% of cases due to compression axial load at the radiocapitellar joint. Avulsion fractures of the medial or lateral epicondyle occur in 12% of cases and fracture of the coronoid process has been noted in 10% of elbow dislocations.

In adolescents, it is sometimes difficult to diagnose fractures of the medial epicondyle (12), which may have intra-articular extension and result in posttraumatic arthritis. Medial epicondylar fractures can also predispose to secondary dislocation as a result of the loss of integrity of the medial collateral ligament (13).

Osteochondral fractures probably occur more often than they are diagnosed, while intra-articular fractures of the capitellum are rare.

Associated injuries at other sites—such as fractures or dislocations of the distal radius (Fig. 3) or ulnar styloid, perilunate dislocations, and shoulder injuries—are found in 12% of elbow dislocations and should always be suspected.

Significant soft tissue swelling leading to high compartmental pressure can compromise the neurovascular structures as well as causing displacement of the bones. Neurological stretch injuries can also be noted.

C. Clinical Evaluation

Elbow dislocation is usually easy to diagnose unless excessive soft tissue swelling complicates it. Physical examination should include neurovascular assessment and evaluation of ipsilateral associated injuries. All injuries should be assessed before reduction is attempted. Neurovascular evaluation before and after reduction should be documented. A case of median nerve entrapment in the ulnohumeral joint has been reported after elbow dislocation. Monitoring of the soft

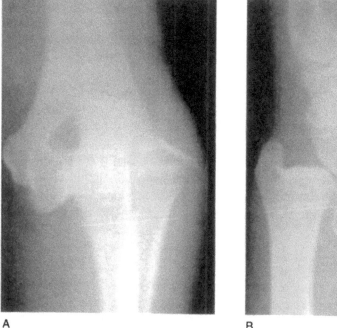
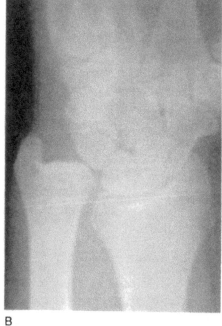

A   B

Figure 3 A. Dislocation of the elbow. B. Associated dislocation of the distal radioulnar joint.

tissue swelling is essential in cases of massive soft tissue injury in order to avoid missing the diagnosis of compartment syndrome.

Radiographic evaluation before and after reduction of is also essential. Anteroposterior, lateral, and oblique views should be taken as routine radiographs. Additional views include radial head, axial, and varus/valgus stress views (Fig. 4), which are usually taken under anesthesia while assessing the associated ligamentous injuries.

After reduction, the elbow should be examined for instability; this is better performed with the patient under general anesthesia. Varus, valgus, and posteolateral rotatory instability is assessed (14). The varus and valgus test is performed with the elbow in extension and 30 degrees of flexion in order to unlock the olecranon from the fossa. The testing should be performed with the forearm in supination, since in pronation instability is prevented with the use of the intact medial soft tissues as a hinge. The anatomical congruity of the ulnohumeral joint is also assessed throughout the entire extension-flexion arc for stability. Posterolateral rotatory instability is diagnosed with the lateral pivot-shift test (2).

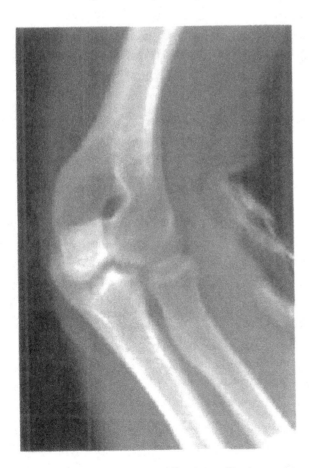

Figure 4   Valgus stress view of the elbow.

III. TREATMENT

The goals of treatment in elbow dislocations are (1) anatomical reduction and restoration of articular alignment without producing further injury, (2) restoration of stability, and (3) short posttraumatic immobilization followed by early mobilization.

In simple dislocations without fracture, the ligamentous injuries usually allow stable reduction of the elbow joint. Nevertheless, due to extensive disruption of the flexor-pronator muscle mass, gross instability after reduction can be noted in simple dislocations (15).

In complex dislocations, acute instability after reduction is not uncommon (14%) and is usually associated with radial head, coronoid, medial, or lateral epicondylar fracture and disruption of the lateral collateral ligament (16).

A. Closed Reduction

Closed reduction of pulled elbow in children includes elbow flexion and forearm supination while the radial head is palpated for reduction. Successful reduction usually permits immediate mobilization.

Closed reduction of posterior simple elbow dislocations can be achieved in some cases even without anesthetic, but this is not advocated, because pain relief and muscle relaxation prevent further injuries during reduction. Also, the assessment of stability after reduction with the patient under anesthetia is much easier and more reliable.

The maneuver for closed reduction consists of manual traction of the forearm in supination with the elbow in a slightly flexed position. An assistant provides countertraction of the humerus. Axial compression of the olecranon with medial or lateral translocation depending on the pattern of the posterior dislocation, and gradual flexion of the elbow is done until reduction is achieved. Initial hyperextension of the elbow may be needed to unlock the coronoid from the distal humerus.

After reduction, the elbow is assessed for stability as previously described; if it is stable, a posterior splint at 90 degrees is applied for 1 week (maximum 10 days). Close observation of the neurovascular status is essential for the first 24–48 h after reduction to assess for possible development of compartment syndrome. After 1 week of immobilization, the splint is discarded and mobilization of the elbow joint begins.

Closed reduction of anterior simple dislocations consist of gentle flexion of the forearm to unlock the olecranon from the trochlea, followed by traction and posterior displacement of the forearm to achieve reduction. Palpitation of the triceps to assess for possible avulsion should always be performed after the reduction.

In case of the rare divergent dislocation, reduction of each bone must be performed separately. Due to rupture of the interosseous ligament, the incidence of postreduction instability is high (8).

Complex elbow dislocations usually require operative treatment to achieve an anatomical and stable reduction.

B. Operative Treatment

Generally, the indication for operative treatment is inability to achieve concentric and stable (even after immobilization for up to 10 days) closed reduction. If the dislocation of the elbow is associated with type II or III radial head or coronoid process fractures or with fracture of the epicondyles, open treatment and assessment of these injuries is recommended, because these factors predispose to elbow instability (17).

In most cases, a lateral approach of the elbow is adequate for open reduction and assessment of instability. Through this approach, any interposed obstacles of concentric reduction, such as soft tissue or osteochondral fractures, can be removed. Disruption of the annular ligament must also be assessed with direct repair or with reconstruction.

Type II fractures of the radial head should be fixed to increase the stability of the reduction. The nonarticulating portion of the radial head is the most common portion to be fractured because it lacks strong subchondral osseous support. Fixation of this fragment can be easily achieved with the insertion of an Arbeitsgemeinschaft für Osteosynthesefragen (AO) miniscrew through the fragment into the main portion of the radial head. Comminuted fractures of the radial head (type III) should be assessed with removal of the fragments and replacement with a titanium radial-head implant providing lateral (valgus) stability to the elbow joint. Occasionally dislocation of the elbow is associated with compressive fracture of the radial neck (18). In this case fixation of the fracture is recommended with the use of an AO miniplate, which is placed at the nonarticulating one-third of the radius, so that pronation and supination are not blocked. Again, fixation of the radial neck provides lateral stability to the elbow joint and allows a possible rupture of the medial collateral ligament to heal. With the stabilization of the lateral column, surgical repair of ruptures of the medial collateral ligament is not necessary. Although some authors (16) advocate repair of the medial collateral ligament, this has not proved to be superior to no repair.

Avulsion fractures of the coronoid process that involves 50% or more of the coronoid process (type II and III) usually affect the stability of the elbow joint after relocation and have to be fixed. The avulsed fragment can be fixed through a medial approach with the elbow in flexion (it is difficult to do so through a lateral approach) with the use of a cannulated miniscrew, suture anchors, or a tunnel and suture technique. If the coronoid process is comminuted and the fragments cannot be reapproximated to the ulna, the coronoid process can be reconstructed from iliac crest bone graft and fixed to the ulna with a screw.

Lateral epicondylar (Fig. 5) and capitellar fractures should also be fixed if they are large enough to cause instability of the relocated elbow. Fixation is achieved through the lateral approach with the use of a cannulated screw or K

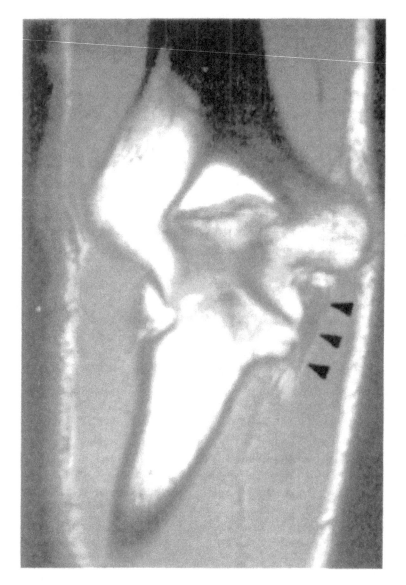

Figure 5   Magnetic resonance imaging (MRI) scan showing avulsion fracture of the lateral epicondyle.

wires. Avulsion fractures of the medial epicondyle are also associated with dislocation of the elbow; if reapproximation after reduction is not adequate, fixation is recommended in order to stabilize the medial ligamentous complex.

In anterior dislocations, the olecranon is usually fractured and fixation is essential to restore reduction and good functional outcome. Previous studies with excision (19) of the proximal olecranon fragment have shown a high incidence of instability.

Acute repair of the lateral ulnar collateral ligament must also be performed if the dislocated elbow remains unstable after reduction. Direct repair can be done with the use of bony anchors if the ligament is avulsed from the humerus or the ulna. If the ligament has a midsubstance tear after direct repair, passing a #2 absorbable suture through the same course as for a ligamentous reconstruction can augment the ligament (Fig. 6). In case of inadequate lateral ligamentous tissue, the ligament can be reconstructed with the use of palmaris longus graft through a lateral approach (Fig. 7). Ruptures of the anterior capsule should also be repaired to increase the stability of the elbow joint.

In our experience, injuries to the medial collateral ligament (Fig. 8) do not have to be repaired. If the elbow remains unstable after fixation of the associated fractures and repair of the lateral collateral ligament and anterior capsule, we recommend the use of an external fixator that will stabilize the joint and allow immediate mobilization. The external fixator is also useful after reconstruction or repair of the ligament or coronoid process because it neutralizes the forces in the joint and allows immediate mobilization (20).

Aggressive surgical treatment for complex dislocations of the elbow will give better results due to increased postreduction stability, allowing early mobilization of the joint and preventing disabling stiffness.

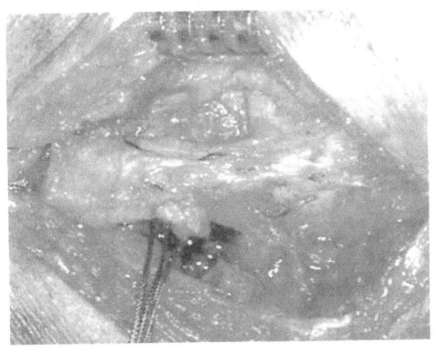

Figure 6   Augmentation of the lateral ulnar collateral ligament (LUCL) repair with a #2 suture.

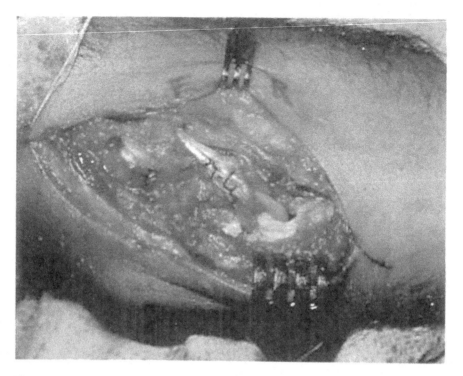

Figure 7 Reconstruction of the LUCL with palmaris longus graft.

IV. COMPLICATIONS

A. Neurovascular

Hyperextension and stretching of the anterior structures may cause spasm, rupture, or thrombosis of the radial artery. Median nerve injuries (21) can also be associated with dislocation of the elbow because of stretching or intra-articular entrapment. Tension of the nerve across the margin of the epicondylar flare can "notch" the bone, producing a late radiographic sign known as Matev's sign (22). Extensive soft tissue injury results in excessive swelling around the elbow, which can lead to a compartment syndrome of the forearm and the development of a Volkman's ischemic syndrome. The ulnar nerve is also in danger during elbow dislocations because of valgus stretching (23). Late cubital tunnel symptoms can also occur due to ossification and scarring within the cubital tunnel.

B. Heterotopic Ossification

Heterotopic ossification can occur (24) in most severe injuries of the elbow. Heterotopic bone formation at the anterior and posterior capsule can dramatically limit the range of motion of the elbow and may need excision. It has been suggested that early excision (between 4 and 12 months) gives better functional

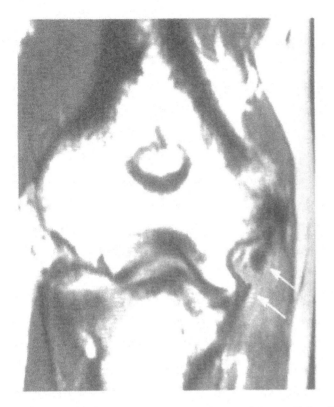

Figure 8   An MRI scan reveals rupture of the medial collateral ligament of the elbow (white arrows).

results than delayed excision. Calcification of the collateral ligaments and myositis ossificans (25) do occur but usually do not restrict elbow motion significantly.

C.   Limited Motion

Limited motion can occur because of capsular thickening, restricting extension more than the flexion. If this is disabling, capsular release is recommended, with aggressive physiotherapy postoperatively and continuous passive motion equipment. Note that in some cases release of soft tissue can produce instability of the elbow.

Osteochondral fractures or articular flakes can also limit motion or produce a locking sensation typical of a loose body. In that case, reoperation and removal of such fragments is recommended. Osteophytes at the posterior or anterior tip of the olecranon (Fig. 9) can limit motion, with pain at the end of the extension/ flexion arc, and may need to be removed.

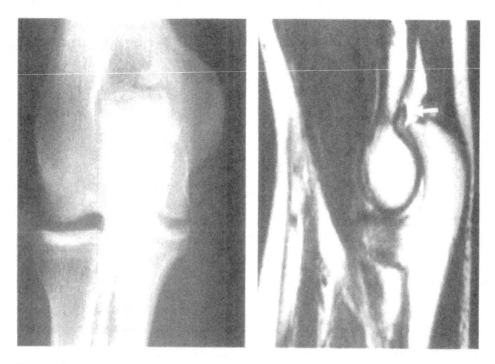

Figure 9   Osteophytes at the olecranon fossa can cause pain or restriction of extension.

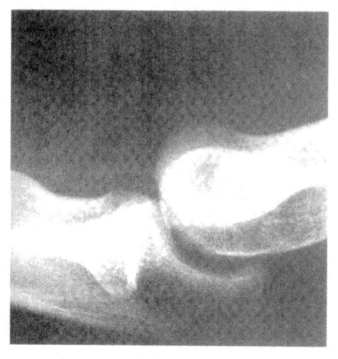

Figure 10   Instability of the elbow in extension 3 months after reduction of a dislocated elbow.

D. Recurrent Instability

Instability is a common complication of elbow dislocations (Fig. 10) and can occur because of insufficient fixation of the bony associated injuries (radial head and coronoid fractures) or insufficient repair of the collateral ligaments (26). The cause should be identified and the patient reoperated on to resolve the problem. Assessment and treatment of recurrent instability is technically demanding.

V. PROGNOSIS

Simple dislocations usually have an excellent outcome with good range of motion and stability and absence of pain. If treated correctly, complex elbow dislocations have a good result in 85% of uncomplicated cases (3,27). Improvement continues after treatment for 6 to 18 months. Immobilization for more than 2 weeks results in elbow contractures with poor functional outcome and thus should be avoided.

REFERENCES

1. JW King, HF Brelsford, HS Tullos. Analysis of the pitching arm of the professional baseball pitcher. Clin Orthop 67:116, 1969.
2. SW O'Driscoll, BF Morrey, S Korinek, KN An. Elbow subluxation and dislocation: A spectrum of instability. Clin Orthop 280:186, 1992.
3. RL Linscheid, DK Wheeler. Elbow dislocations. JAMA 194:1171, 1965.
4. JO Sojberg, P Helmig, P Kjaerrsgaard-Anderson. Dislocation of the elbow: An experimental study of the ligamentous injuries. Orthopedics 12(3):461, 1989.
5. DP Boyete, HC Ahoski, AH London. Subluxation of the head of the radius—"nursmaid's elbow." J Pediatr 32:278, 1948.
6. JC Delee. Transverse divergent dislocation of the elbow in a child. J Bone Joint Surg 63A:322, 1981.
7. DJ Blatz. Anterior dislocation of the elbow. Findings in a case of Ehlers-Danlos syndrome. Orthop Rev 10:129, 1981.
8. JL Holbrook, NE Green. Divergent pediatric elbow dislocation: A case report. Clin Orthop 234:72, 1988.
9. JP O'Hara, BF Morrey, EW Johnson, KA Johnson. Dislocations and fractured dislocations of the elbow. Fracture Conference. Minn Med 58:697, 1975.
10. D Scharplatz, M Allgower. Fracture dislocations of the elbow. Injury 7:143, 1975.
11. DN Smith, JR Lee. The radiological diagnosis of posttraumatic effusion of the elbow joint nad its clinical significance. Injury 10:115, 1978.
12. AA Tayob, RA Shively. Bilateral elbow dislocations intraarticular displacement of the medial epicondyles. J Trauma 20:332, 1980.
13. DW Purser. Dislocation of the elbow and inclusion of the medial epicondyle in the adult. J Bone Joint Surg 36B:247, 1954.
14. SW O'Driscoll. Instability. Hand Clin 10:405, 1994.
15. HS Tullos, JB Bennett, D Shepard. Elbow instability in the adult. AAOS. In: Instructional Course Lectures. St Louis: Mosby, 1986, p 59.

16. O Josefsson, C Gentz, D Johnell, B Wenderberg. Surgical versus non-surgical treatment of ligamentous injuries following dislocation of the elbow joint. J Bone Joint Surg 69A:605, 1987.
17. BF Morrey. Complex instability of the elbow. J Bone Joint Surg 79A:460, 1997.
18. BF Morrey. Current concepts in the treatment of fractures of the radial head, the olecranon, and the coronoid. J Bone Joint Surg 77A:316, 1995.
19. JS Nevasier, J Winckstrom. Dislocation of the elbow: A retrospective study of 115 patients. South Med J, 70:172, 1977.
20. BF Morrey, KN An. Articular ligamentous contributions to the stability of the elbow joint. Am J Sports Med 11:315, 1983.
21. KA Galbraith, CJ McCullogh. Acute nerve injury as a complication of closed fractures or dislocations of the elbow. Injury 11:159, 1979.
22. I Matev. A radiological sign of entrapment of the median nerve in the elbow joint after posterior dislocation: A report of two cases. J Bone Joint Surg 48B:353, 1976.
23. RK Scharma, NA Covelle. An unsual ulnar nerve injury associated with dislocation of the elbow. Injury 8:145, 1976.
24. G Hait, JA Boswick, NH Stone. Heterotopic bone formation secondary to trauma. J Trauma 10:405, 1970.
25. HC Thompson, A Garcia. Myositis ossificans (aftermath of elbow injury). Clin Orthop 50:129, 1967.
26. D Ring, JB Jupiter. Reconstruction of posttraumatic instability. Clin Orthop 370:44, 2000.
27. TL Melhoff, PC Noble, JB Bennett, HS Tullos. Simple dislocation of the elbow in the adult. J Bone Joint Surg 70A:244, 1988.

2

Treatment of Soft Tissue Injuries About the Upper Extremity

Robert J. Goitz and Brian M. Jurbala
University of Pittsburgh Medical Center, Pittsburgh, Pennsylvania, U.S.A.

I. INTRODUCTION

Trauma involving the upper extremity may result in soft tissue injuries that have a greater impact on the ultimate outcome than the associated fracture or dislocation. For instance, an ulnar nerve injury associated with an elbow fracture/dislocation can result in a decrease of 50 and 75% of grip and pinch strength, respectively (1). Therefore, appropriate diagnosis and management of all soft tissue injuries associated with upper extremity trauma is paramount to obtain an optimal outcome.

This chapter outlines the management of injuries of the soft tissues involving nerves, tendons, muscle, and skin.

II. NERVE INJURIES

A. General Considerations

Due to the relatively subcutaneous position of the neurovascular structures of the arm and their anatomical proximity to the bones in this region, they are susceptible to injury with blunt trauma, fractures, dislocations, and penetrating soft tissue injuries. The majority of closed injuries are neuropraxias and recover in time (2). Higher-energy injuries associated with open fractures or dislocations have less chance of spontaneous recovery (3). The overall functional recovery of the extremity will be significantly affected by the degree of nerve recovery. Therefore nerve injuries associated with upper extremity trauma should be diagnosed early and properly treated.

B. Anatomy

A fundamental knowledge of the basic anatomy of the peripheral nerve is necessary to undertake a successful repair (Fig. 1). The outer shell of the peripheral nerve, or epineurium, is responsible for cushioning the nerve fascicles and relieving tension with longitudinal traction. The perineurium surrounds individual nerve fascicles, and is a peripheral extension of the blood-brain barrier. It helps to maintain a homeostatic environment for the nerve fibers by acting as a diffusion barrier. Within each fascicle are groups of individual axons surrounded by collagenous tissue or endoneurium; this acts as packing between the axons and participates in the formation of the Schwann cell tube, or endoneurial tube.

C. Classification

Nerve injuries are classified according to the Sunderland classification (4). In grade I injuries (neuropraxias), the nerve sustains a focal demyelination affecting axonal transport but the structural integrity of the individual axons and nerve remains intact. Walllerian degeneration does not occur, there is no Tinel's sign, and complete recovery is expected within weeks to months. In grade II injuries (axonotomesis), the axon is disrupted but the endoneurium remains intact. Wallarian degeneration occurs distal to the injury and a Tinel's sign can be used to follow axon regeneration, which occurs at a rate of approximately 1 to 2 mm per day.

In grade III injuries, there is increased destruction to the internal architecture of the nerve, which ultimately leads to increased internal scarring and less chance for useful recovery. Grade IV injuries are characterized by a neuroma in continuity and grade V injuries (neurotomesis) are marked by complete transection of the nerve trunk with no chance of recovery without surgical repair.

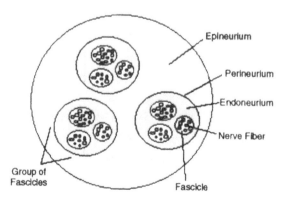

Figure 1   Cross sectional diagram of a typical peripheral nerve.

D. Diagnosis

Any patient with significant trauma about the arm should undergo a thorough sensory and motor examination evaluating the function of the radial, posterior interosseous, median, anterior interosseous, and ulnar nerves. Serial examinations are often required following closed injuries to assess spontaneous recovery or the possible need for surgical intervention.

Electrodiagnostic studies are usually not useful in the early postinjury period (<3 weeks) (5). In the case of closed injuries, a baseline study performed at 3 weeks postinjury may detect denervation changes in muscle and slowing of conduction velocity. Reinnervation potentials are usually evident by 8 weeks and can, along with an advancing Tinel's sign and improving motor function on clinical examination, support the expectant management of these closed injuries. Continued evidence of denervation—such as positive sharp waves and persistent fibrillation potentials on electromyography (EMG)—indicates ongoing nerve dysfunction and may support early operative exploration.

E. Treatment

There are common nerve injuries that occur with specific fractures, such as a radial nerve injury with the Holstein-Lewis humeral shaft fracture (6), a posterior interosseous nerve injury with a Monteggia fracture/dislocation (7), and an anterior interosseous nerve injury with a supracondylar humeral fracture (8). These specific patterns of injury and their treatment algorithms are detailed elsewhere in the text. In general, however, most of these nerve injuries, when associated with a closed fracture or dislocation that is otherwise treated in a closed fashion, can be followed with serial examinations and a baseline electrodiagnostic study at 3 to 4 weeks postinjury. If there is no evidence of nerve regeneration, either by examination or electrodiagnostic tests by 2 to 3 months, exploration is warranted. The decision for operative exploration should be made no later than 6 months postinjury so as to allow for axonal regrowth in a timely fashion prior to motor endplate degeneration and subsequent muscle fibrosis (9).

Nerve injuries associated with open fractures or penetrating trauma warrant operative exploration of the involved nerve, since these injuries are associated with nerve transection and a low probability of spontaneous recovery without operative management (6). Early repair may optimize the ultimate return of function and minimize prolonged disability.

1. Techniques of Nerve Repair

Preparation.   The patient's limb should be exsanguinated to produce a bloodless field. Dissection and mobilization of the individual nerve stumps should precede any attempt at repair under high-powered loupe magnification or with the help of a microscope. Transposition of the damaged nerve, such as the ulnar nerve at the cubital tunnel, will not only minimize tension on the repair but move the nerve out of the scarred bed and minimize adhesions during the recovery period. The ends of the nerve are then sharply transected with a #11 blade over a tongue depressor back to normal-appearing fascicles. This step is critical to minimize scar at the repair site.

Primary Versus Secondary Nerve Repair. The laboratory and clinical results of primary repair (within hours of the injury) appear to be superior to those from secondary repair (greater than 1 week postinjury) when the wound is clean, well vascularized, and sharply transected with a repair under minimal tension (11). However, if the injury does not allow for primary repair due to excessive contamination or for other reasons, the nerve ends should be tagged to facilitate later identification and secondary repair.

2. End-to-End Nerve Repair

When a peripheral nerve is transected sharply, Wallerian degeneration will take place in the distal stump, leaving the endoneurial framework intact. The only remnant of nerve fiber remaining is the basement membrane or Schwann cell tube filled with Schwann cells. A properly aligned end-to-end repair must therefore oppose the corresponding endoneurial tubes in order for neurotization to occur. The techniques available include a direct end-to-end anastomosis with an epineurial repair or a group fascicular repair. The results of primary repair with epineurial suture techniques are nearly equivalent and more easily accomplished than results from group or individual fasicular repair techniques (12).

Epineurial repair is accomplished by trimming the nerve stumps perpendicular to the long axis of the nerve and aligning the nerve using both vascular landmarks and the topography of fascicular groups within the nerve as a guide. An incongruous repair will result in fascicular malalignment and bulging at the repair site, leading to the formation of a neuroma, incomplete neurotization, and an inferior functional outcome. An epineural repair of a peripheral nerve using 8-0 nylon suture is best done under a microscope or with loupe magnifiation (Fig. 2).

Nerve Grafting. If a tensionless repair is not possible, nerve grafting may be considered. The sural nerve provides a readily accessible means of 30 to 40 cm

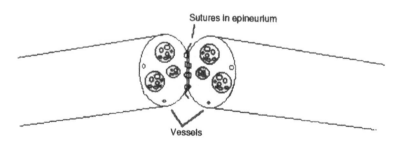

Figure 2 Diagram of epineural repair while aligning perivascular vessels and intraneural fasicular groups.

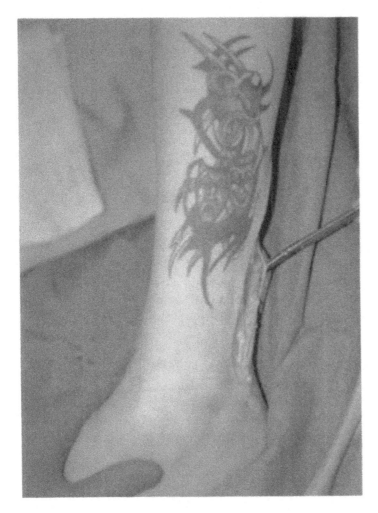

Figure 3   Harvest site of sural nerve graft between lateral malleolus and Achilles tendon.

of nerve graft with relatively low morbidity. For larger defects, the graft can be harvested from its origin at the sciatic nerve in the popliteal fossa or, if shorter segments will suffice, harvesting can begin at the posterior lateral malleolus and be dissected proximally as needed (Fig. 3). If the diameter of the recipient nerve exceeds that of the sural nerve, cable grafting can be undertaken with multiple short segments of the sural nerve combined into a larger diameter (Fig. 4). The orientation of the sural nerve should be reversed to minimize the loss of branches along its length.

III.   TENDON INJURIES

Tendon lacerations should be anticipated with any deep wound about the upper extremity. A sharp laceration through the triceps, biceps, or forearm tendons

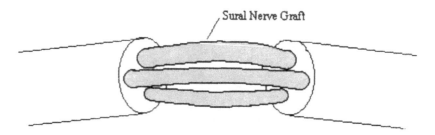

Figure 4   Diagram of cable sural nerve graft bridging nerve defect.

should be repaired acutely. After the tendon edges are debrided, a suture of an appropriate gauge is used with a "Kessler type" core stitch to secure the tendon edges (Fig. 5). The suture caliber depends on the tendon size and relative tension of the repair. Digital flexor or extensor tendons lacerated in the forearm are generally repaired with 3-0 nonabsorbable braided sutures. Wrist flexor or extensor tendons are repaired with 2-0 sutures. The biceps and triceps may be repaired with 0 sutures. Tendon avulsions can be repaired using suture anchors secured with a core suture.

After tendon repair, the extremity is generally immobilized in a position to minimize the tension on the repaired muscle/tendon unit. If digital flexor tendons are repaired, passive mobilization of the digits is initiated as soon as soft tissue healing allows. Lacerations of the digital extensor tendons require immobilization of the metacarpophalangeal joints in extension for 3 weeks. Generally, active range of motion of adjacent joints is initiated at 3 to 4 weeks after repair. Strengthening is initiated at approximately 8 weeks postrepair.

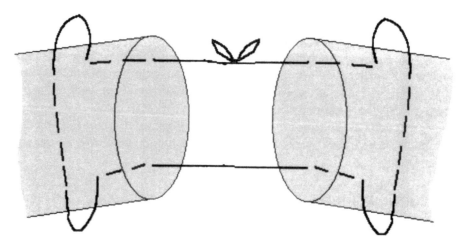

Figure 5   Kessler repair with single core stitch in tendon.

IV.   MUSCLE LACERATIONS

Lacerations of muscle bellies should also be treated aggressively. After debridement of the nonviable or contaminated edges, the muscle may be repaired with a slow-dissolving absorbable suture. Large figure-of-eight sutures may be placed through the muscle to reapproximate the edges. The fascia should not be repaired alone, since this will not restore the length of tissue that is required to provide maximal force production. Postrepair therapy is similar to that outlined above (Sec. III) in the discussion of tendon repair.

V.   COVERAGE OF SOFT TISSUE DEFECTS

A.   General Considerations

Open injuries of the upper extremity require the clinician to perform a thorough examination for muscle/tendon and nerve function, traversing the injured site. The neurological evaluation should include an assessment of two-point discrimination to diagnose not only major nerve injuries but also sensory nerve dysfunction. The choice of coverage to a wound may be affected by possible future surgeries, such as tendon transfers, repairs, or nerve grafts. For example, if it were known that a patient would require tendon transfers to restore flexor tendon function, a skin graft would not be adequate over the volar forearm due to the resulting scarring. A fasciocutaneous flap might be optimal to allow for adequate excursion of the transferred tendons.

Low-velocity open injuries can often be adequately treated with a one-stage debridement and repair of damaged structures, followed by the necessary coverage. High-energy injuries require multiple debridements to determine tissue viability.

The decision on the optimal type of tissue coverage for a wound defect relies heavily on an assessment of the wound bed. Healthy muscle and fat provide the optimal bed for a skin graft. Exposed tendons can be skin grafted if the paratenon is not violated. Although exposed bone with an intact periosteum can be skin grafted, this is not optimal due to the resultant adhesions and lack of mobility of the healed skin, which often limits motion and is persistently painful. In addition, although the antecubital fossa is covered with muscle, a skin graft in this area will often limit motion and result in a suboptimal outcome. Soft tissue coverage over joints must be mobile and is more optimally achieved with a fasciocutaneous local rotation or regional flap such as a radial forearm flap, which is described below.

B.   Secondary Intention

Wound healing by secondary intention requires a clean, healthy bed devoid of stripped bone, tendon, nerves, or an exposed joint. The size of the wound affects mainly the healing time. Even large wounds will eventually heal with a linear scar. Healing by secondary intention requires frequent dressing changes, which may not be optimal if a cast is required for added stability to an unstable fracture or dislocation.

The first stage of wound healing is a local inflammatory response. Local blood vessels dilate and an exudate forms, which includes a fibrin clot and inflammatory cells. Phagocytosis of necrotic tissue occurs and fibroblasts begin to produce scar to bridge the defect. Epithelial cells multiply and the scar tissue contracts, ultimately to decrease the size of the wound (13).

Wet-to-dry dressing changes with normal saline three times a day is fairly standard treatment; however, numerous methods yielding similar results have been described. The wet-to-dry dressing changes with gauze enhance debridement of necrotic tissue to obtain a healthy tissue bed and lessen the phagocytic load. Once a "beefy red" granulation tissue is obtained, a less abrasive moist protective covering such as Xeroform (Kendall Sherwood, Mansfield, MA) may be used once or twice a day.

The recent availability of the Vacuum-Assisted Wound Closure (VAC) system (Kinetic Concepts, Inc., San Antonio, TX) has expanded the indications for healing by secondary intention. Less than optimal wound beds may be treated with the VAC system to induce granulation tissue more expediently (14). A negative pressure is applied to the wound through a sealed, open-cell foam dressing. The VAC system stimulates the granulation tissue by removing excess fluid, increasing local blood flow, and enhancing debridement of the wound. Considering that the VAC system requires a machine hookup 24 h per day, the authors have found it more useful in lower extremity trauma, where patients are often not ambulatory. For upper extremity wounds, it is mostly used in patients with a marginal wound bed with poor options for adjacent tissue advancement who are not candidates for free tissue coverage.

C. Skin Grafts

Split-thickness skin grafts may be optimal over exposed muscle or fat, such as the proximal forearm or arm. Considering that skin grafts heal by adhering to the tissues below, tissue mobility is a major consideration. If future surgery is required below the area to be skin-grafted, there is a higher probability of a suboptimal result. Skin-grafted areas may be more prone to wound breakdown and tendon adherence.

Potential donor sites include the lateral thigh, buttocks, and abdomen, since these areas provide thick skin with minimal donor-site morbidity. On average, a thickness of 0.016 to 0.018 in. is taken from the donor site using a dermatome. Thinner grafts of 0.012 to 0.014 in. are taken in elderly or very young patients. The skin graft is generally meshed at the ratio of 1:1.5 to allow for drainage from under the graft. Unmeshed grafts are more esthetic but require a very dry recipient site and pose a higher risk of incomplete healing due to the development of a hematoma or seroma from under the graft.

D. Rotation Flaps

Rotation flaps are random-pattern flaps that make use of normal adjacent tissue to close both the donor site and recipient site. The defect site must be relatively small, less than 3 cm in the arm, with mobile healthy adjacent skin. However, following trauma, the adjacent skin is often suboptimal due to extension of the zone of injury. Experience in evaluating tissues for future viability, especially when they are incised for transfer, is paramount in choosing a rotation flap to minimize the possibility of increasing the defect site by rotating a flap that ultimately necroses.

Rotation flaps are ideally used for triangular defects. The flap is developed as an extension of the widest edge of the triangle in a curvilinear direction, as illustrated in Fig. 6A. The flap is developed in the suprafascial avascular plane just above the sensory nerves. Because the arm and forearm have such a rich vascularity, a 2:1 ratio is often adequate to avoid ischemia if minimal tension is placed on the edges of the flap. A back cut (Fig. 6B) or Burrow's triangle (Fig. 6C) may be used to facilitate advancement of the flap. This moves the pivot point closer to the defect but also increases the length-to-width ratio and the risk of ischemia (13).

E. Transposition Flaps

Lister defined a transposition flap as local tissue that "is raised from its bed and moved laterally either to an immediately adjacent defect or over a peninsula of intervening skin" (15). Such a flap is commonly used to cover the olecranon by using skin from the volar or dorsal forearm, which has a healthy muscle in its bed that can be safely skin-grafted. Lister's simple transposition flap is illustrated in Fig. 7, with subsequent modifications to improve mobility but minimize tension in

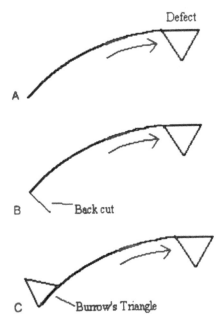

Figure 6 A. Diagram of rotation flap. B. Back cut. C. Burrow's triangle.

Defect

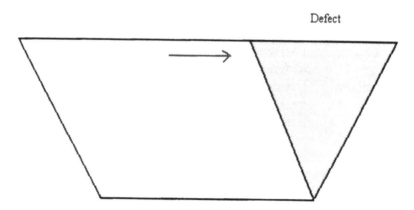

Figure 7   Diagram of a transposition flap.

the flap. This flap can often be used to close moderate-sized defects in the arm or forearm of approximately 3 to 5 cm using nontraumatized adjacent tissue.

F. Regional Flaps

1.   Radial Forearm Flap

A proximally based radial forearm flap is a versatile fasciocutaneous flap that can be used to cover large defects about the distal humerus, elbow, or proximal forearm (Fig. 8) (16,17). The entire volar forearm skin, subcutaneous tissues, and fascia are supplied by the radial artery through intermuscular perforators found between the brachioradialis and flexor carpi radialis muscles. An Allen's test must be performed preoperatively to ensure a competent arch in the hand. Donor defects up to 6 cm can often be closed primarily on the volar forearm. The skin from the entire volar forearm can be used for the flap, and the donor site can be safely skin-grafted as long as the paratenon is maintained on the volar flexor tendons. An intact paratenon will allow for adequate nutrition of the skin graft and ensure tendon mobility. The forearm donor site can be esthetically displeasing, which must be discussed with the patient.

2.   Posterior Interosseous Artery Flap

This is also a fasciocutaneous flap that can cover defects similar to those covered by the radial forearm flap. Its main indication is for injuries that require regional flap coverage about the elbow when the radial forearm flap is not available.

The posterior interosseous artery (PIOA) is a branch of the ulnar artery that supplies dorsal skin via septal perforators between the extensor carpi ulnaris and extensor digiti minimi (18). The axis of the PIOA is centered on a line drawn from the lateral epicondyle to the dorsal radioulnar joint at the wrist. Flap elevation is similar to that of the radial artery flap but more demanding (Fig. 9).

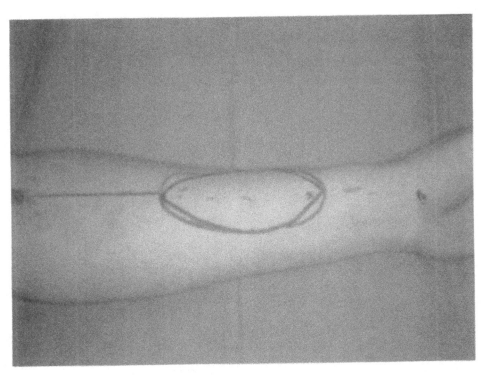

Figure 8 Radial forearm flap (elbow on the left with the radial artery inflow indicated by the solid line).

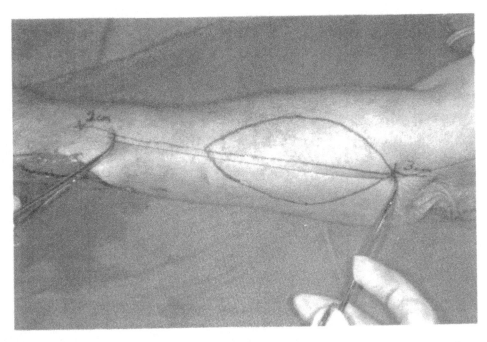

Figure 9 Posterior interosseous artery flap drawn distally-based to cover an ulnar hand defect (elbow on the right).

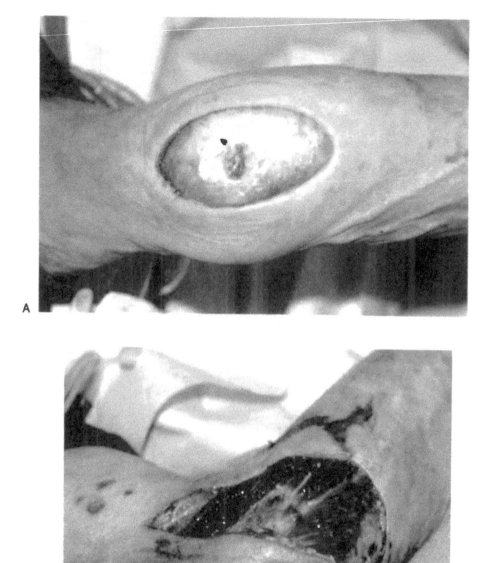

Figure 10   A. Olecranon wound (hand on the right). B. Extended lateral arm flap used to cover the olecranon defect.

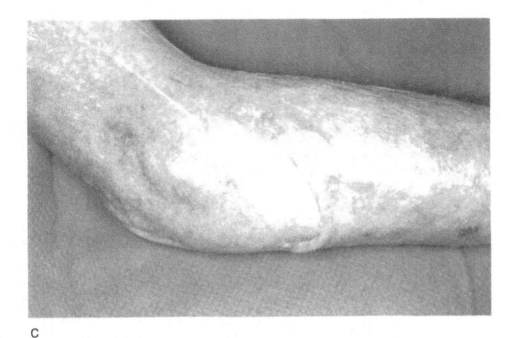

C

Figure 10   C. Final appearance.

3.   Extended Lateral Arm Flap

The standard lateral arm flap is based on the posterior radial collateral artery, a terminal branch of the profunda brachii found at the lateral intermuscular septum of the distal arm (19). This vessel continues along the dorsal forearm in line with the brachioradialis and supplies skin up to 18 cm distal to the lateral epicondyle. This flap can be successfully used to cover posterior or anterior elbow defects up to 5 cm in width (Fig. 10).

4.   Pedicled Latissimus Dorsi Flap

The latissimus dorsi muscle at times may provide optimal coverage to defects of the arm, elbow, and forearm up to 10 cm distal to the olecranon (20). Its main advantage is that it is well outside the zone of injury and is quite reliable in its blood supply from the thoracodorsal artery in the axilla. Its use results in minimal functional and cosmetic deficits. In addition, it may be used to restore elbow flexor or extensor function while also providing tissue coverage (Fig. 11).

VI.   CONCLUSION

Upper extremity trauma often results in injuries to multiple tissues, often requiring individualized treatment. A knowledge of the timing and treatment options for each individual tissue will ultimately result in a better outcome. The treating trauma surgeon should not ignore associated soft tissue injuries even in cases of

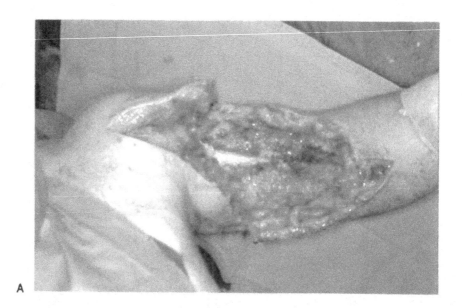

A

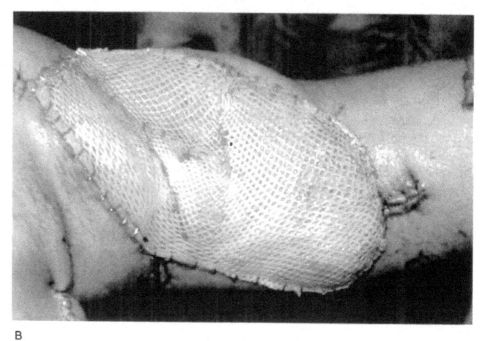

B

Figure 11 A. Anterior arm defect with loss of triceps and exposed humeral plate (shoulder on left). B. Pedicled latissimus dorsi muscle flap used to provide coverage for the open humeral fracture but also for reanimation of elbow flexion.

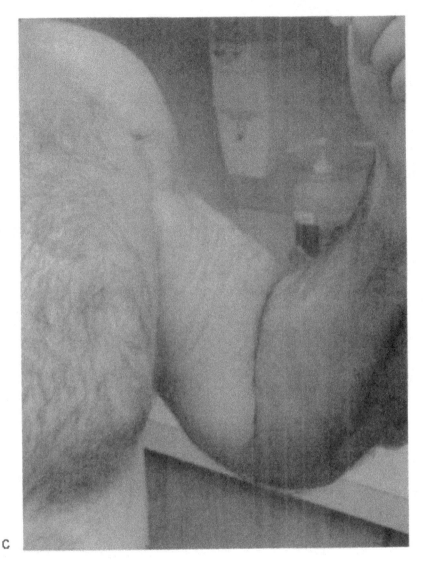

C

Figure 11   C. Final follow-up appearance.

severe bone and joint injuries. The ultimate outcome and prognosis for the patient will often depend more on the associated nerve or tendon injuries than the obvious skeletal abnormality. A coordinated effort between the trauma surgeon and microsurgeon early in the treatment course is recommended.

REFERENCES

1. L Mannerfelt. Studies on the hand in ulnar nerve paralysis. A clinical-experimental investigation in normal and anomalous innervation. Acta Orthop Scand Suppl 87: 89–97, 1996.

2. FH Pollock, D Drake, EG Bovill, L Day, PG Trefton. Treatment of radial neuropathy associated with fractures of the humerus. J Bone Joint Surg 63A:239–243, 1981.

3. GE Omer Jr. Results of interested peripheral nerve injuries. Clin Orthop 163:15–19, 1982.

4. S Sunderland. A classification of peripheral nerve injuries producing loss of function. Brain 74L:491–516, 1951.

5. C Bufalini, G Pescatori. Posterior cervical electromyography in the diagnosis and prognosis of brachial plexus injuries. J Bone Joint Surg 51B:627, 1969.

6. A Holstein, GB Lewis. Fractures of the humerus with radial lnerve paralysis. J Bone Joint Surg 45A:1382–1388, 1963.

7. P Jessing. Monteggia lesions and their complicating nerve damage. Acta Orthop Scand. 46:601, 1975.

8. SJ Mubarek, CD Wallace. Complications of supracondylar fractures of the elbow. In: Morrey BF, ed. The Elbow and Its Disorders. Philadelphia: W. B. Saunders, 2000, pp 201–218.

9. S Sutherland. Capacity of reinnervated muscles to function efficiently after prolonged denervation. Arch Neurol Psychiatry 64:755–771, 1950.

10. HJ Seddon. Nerve lesions complicating certain closed bone injuries. JAMA 135: 691–694, 1947.

11. R Birch, ARM Raji. Repair of median and ulnar nerve. Primary suture is best. J Bone Joint Surg 73B:154–157, 1991.

12. EFSW Wilgis. Techniques of epineural and group fascicular repair. In: Gelberman R (ed), Operative Nerve Repair & Reconstruction. Philadelphia: Lippincott, 1991, pp 287–295.

13. RJ Goitz, JG Westkemper, MM Tomaino, DG Sotereanos. Soft tissue defects of the digits: Coverage considerations. In: Moy OJ, ed. Hand Clinics. Philadelphia: W. B. Saunders, 1997, pp 189–205.

14. JF Mooney, LC Argenta, MW Marks, MJ Morykwas, AJ DeFranco. Treatment of soft tissue defects in pediatric patients using the VAC system. Clin Orthop 376: 26–31, 2000.

15. GD Lister, T Gibson. Closure of rhomboid skin defects: The flaps of Limber and Dufourmental. Br J Plast Surg 25:300–314, 1972.

16. RJ Goitz, MM Tomaino. Regional flaps. In: Fitzgerald R, Kaufer H, Malkani A, eds. Mosby, Orthopaedics. St Louis: 2002, pp 1803–1807.

17. G Foucher, F Van Genechten, F Merle, et al. A compound radial artery forearm flap in hand surgery: An original modification of the Chinese forearm flap. Br J Plastic Surg 37:139–148, 1984.

18. CV Pendato, AC Maspuelet, JP Chevrel. The anatomic basis of the fasciocutaneous flap of the posterior interosseous artery. Surg Radiol Anat 8:209–215, 1986.

19. RG Meirer, C Schrank, R Putz. Posterior radial collateral artery as the basis of the lateral forearm flap. J Reconstr Microsurg 16:21–25, 2000.

20. M Stevanovic, F Sharpe, JM Itamura. Treatment of soft tissue problems about the elbow. Clin Orthop 371:127–137, 2000.

3

Fractures of the Forearm

Kevin J. Pugh
The Ohio State University, Columbus, Ohio, U.S.A.

I. ANATOMY

The forearm—through the elbow, the wrist, and both radioulnar joints—facilitates positioning of the hand in space. This, in turn, facilitates positioning of the upper extremity to accomplish the activities of daily living.

The radius and ulna function as a ring, connected through the proximal and distal radioulnar joints. Like all ring structures, it is difficult to break it in just one place. Thus, injuries to one portion of the ring should prompt the examiner to be diligent in ruling out injuries to other parts of the ring. The ring comprises more than the radius and ulna, and not all parts are bony. The proximal radioulnar joint is bounded by the elbow capsule and the annular ligament. The distal radioulnar joint is bounded by the wrist capsule, dorsal and volar radioulnar ligaments, fibrocartilaginous articular disc, and triangular fibrocartilage complex.

The proximal end of the ulna consists of the olecranon and coronoid processes. Together, these form the articular surface of the ulnohumeral joint. The olecranon, which lies in a subcutaneous position, is especially vulnerable to direct trauma. The proximal ulnohumeral joint allows motion only in the anteroposterior plane and functions as a hinge for elbow flexion and extension. The triceps inserts broadly on the posterior surface of the olecranon process. Fractures of the olecranon process disrupt not only the articular surface of the ulnohumeral joint but also the insertion of the powerful triceps muscle and thus active elbow extension.

At its proximal end, the radius consists of the disc-shaped head, the neck, and the radial tuberosity. The radial head and neck lie within the elbow joint itself. The shallow concavity of the radial head articulates with the capitellum of the distal humerus. Though it flexes and extends with the forearm, it is responsible mainly for the forearm's rotational movement. The head of the radius also articulates with the lateral side of the coronoid process of the ulna to form the proximal radioulnar joint. The annular ligament, whose fibers are intimately associated with the elbow capsule, encircles the radial neck. Though it securely maintains the proximal radioulnar joint, the annular ligament allows the radius full rotation about the ulna. The radial tuberosity, which does not lie within the elbow joint, serves as the insertion point of the powerful biceps tendon, the main supinator of the forearm.

The ulna is a relatively straight bone and functions as a strut about which the radius rotates during normal motion. The radius, the more complex bone of the two, rotates about the ulna to give appropriate pronation and supination. The radial bow is essential for this normal motion, and its reconstruction is a central goal in the treatment of forearm injury (1). The interosseous membrane or ligament, whose fibers run obliquely between the radius and the ulna, is a primary stabilizer and main longitudinal support of the radius (2). Its function is essential in preventing longitudinal migration of the radius should the proximal radius be injured and become length unstable. Injuries to the interosseous membrane can disrupt both proximal and distal radioulnar relationships.

The muscles that cross the forearm create forces that deform the fracture fragments. The radius and ulna are joined by three muscles—the supinator, pronator teres, and pronator quadratus—which insert and originate on the bones of the forearm. In addition to their named function, these muscles, when there is a fracture, bring the radius and ulna closer together and decrease the interosseous space. Muscles that originate on the ulnar side of the forearm and insert on the radial side of the hand exert a pronating force. Muscles that originate on the ulna and interosseous membrane and insert onto the radial side of the dorsum of the wrist exert a supinating force. In addition, the biceps is a powerful supinator of the radius; thus, fractures that occur in the proximal third of forearm are supinated by the powerful pull of this muscle. A thorough knowledge of the muscular anatomy is essential to successful closed management of forearm fractures.

If satisfactory results are to be achieved in fractures of the forearm, it is imperative not only to restore the length of each bone but also to ensure the rotation of each bone, the complex three-dimensional bow of the radius, and the integrity of both radioulnar joints. These must be anatomically reconstructed to maintain proper forearm function. For these reasons, the mainstay of treatment of fractures of the forearm involves open reduction and stable internal fixation.

II. OLECRANON FRACTURES

Fractures of the olecranon occur in response to direct impact to the posterior surface of the elbow, falls onto the flexed elbow, and other falls on the upper extremity that indirectly load the joint. Powerful firing of the triceps muscle can result in an avulsion fracture of the tip of the olecranon process. In general, the distal humerus remains articulated with the intact distal ulnar fragment, while the olecranon fracture fragment is displaced posteriorly and superiorly.

Almost all fractures of the olecranon process are intraarticular. Fractures of the olecranon are thus associated with a bloody effusion in the elbow joint. There may be pain and swelling over the olecranon, and the fracture line may be palpable on the subcutaneous border of the ulna. Most importantly, most patients with an olecranon fracture, as the result of a discontinuity in the triceps mechanism, will have lost the ability to extend the forearm against gravity.

Colton (3) classified olecranon fractures into two major groups: nondisplaced fractures and displaced fractures. A nondisplaced fracture is defined as having less than 2 mm of separation, with no increase in displacement with flexion of the elbow to 90 degrees, and the patient being able to extend the elbow against gravity. Displaced fractures were further subdivided into avulsion fractures, oblique and transverse fractures, comminuted fractures, and those associated with a fracture/dislocation of the elbow. Avulsion fractures result in the separation of a small proximal segment of the olecranon process from the rest of the ulna. With a transverse injury, the fracture line runs obliquely, starting near the deepest portion of the olecranon fossa and emerging on the subcutaneous crest of the proximal part of the ulna. This fracture may either be simple or have more than one fragment. Comminuted fractures have multiple fragments and usually result from direct trauma to the posterior aspect of the elbow. There may be articular impaction and other associated injuries at the elbow. In fracture/dislocations, the olecranon fracture is usually at the distal end and exits near the coronoid process, so that the elbow is unstable as well. This is usually associated with an anterior dislocation of the radius and ulna.

Nondisplaced fractures can be effectively treated by immobilization. Splinting, casting, or bracing of the elbow in 90 degrees of flexion usually results in a satisfactory result. Radiographs must be obtained 7 to 10 days into this treatment to make sure that no displacement has occurred. If displacement occurs, there is still adequate time before healing to effect a successful reconstruction before healing becomes too advanced. Protected range-of-motion exercises can be started at 3 to 4 weeks. Care should be taken to avoid forcible flexion past 90 degrees or resistive exercises until the fracture shows signs of radiographic union.

Displaced fractures of the olecranon are treated operatively. The goals of treatment are to maintain active elbow extension, avoid incongruity of the joint surface, restore elbow stability, and maintain range of motion. Fixation should be achieved with a method that will allow range of motion of the fracture as soon as possible.

Fractures of the olecranon are approached directly from the posterior aspect of the arm. The patient can thus be positioned supine with the arm draped across a stack of towels on the chest, in the lateral position with the arm draped over an arm holder or stack of blankets, or in the prone position using a humeral arm holder. The supine position requires an assistant to constantly hold the arm, while the lateral and prone positions allow the surgeon to operate independently. In multiply injured patients and those with spine injuries, the supine position may be helpful in avoiding further patient compromise.

Avulsion fractures can be intra- or extraarticular. They occur commonly in the elderly population but still require operative treatment in order to restore elbow function. The mainstay of treatment is direct repair of the triceps and proximal fragment to the remaining ulna with nonabsorbable suture through drill holes. The fracture is exposed directly via a posterior approach. A large (#2 or #5) suture is woven through the triceps tendon and then passed through drill holes created in the proximal ulna. Care must be taken to tension the suture with the arm in full extension to have the tightest repair. This method may be supplemented by a tension-band wire (as detailed below) to neutralize the pull of the triceps.

Transverse and short oblique are the most common types of fracture; the tension-band wire technique is the workhorse method for stabilizing these injuries (4). In this method, after fracture reduction, a wire loop is placed around the proximal fragment and through the distal fragment, dorsal to the midaxis of the ulna. In this position, the tensile deforming force of the triceps is neutralized and converted into a compressive force at the fracture site. Improved alignment and greater stability can be provided by introducing two parallel K wires across the fracture site before applying the tension band. This method provides immediate stability and allows early active range of motion.

In the tension-band technique, the fracture site is approached directly from the posterior aspect of the forearm. The fracture site is debrided of clot and soft tissue and reduced anatomically. During reduction, any depressed areas of the joint are elevated, and the fracture is bone-grafted if needed. Two parallel K wires are then placed from dorsal and proximal on the ulna to anterior and distal just across the fracture site. The wires are made long enough to just catch the anterior cortex of the ulna.

Proper placement of the wire loop is essential to the success of this technique. A hole is drilled transversely in the ulna, dorsal to the midaxis of the shaft and distal to the fracture line. As a rule, the distance between the ulnar drill hole and the fracture should be at least equal to the distance from the fracture to the tip of the olecranon. This wire loop is passed deep to the triceps tendon and held in place by the two K wires, bent into a figure-of-eight fashion, and passed through the drill hole. With the forearm in extension, the loop is then tightened and the fracture line compressed. The K wires are then bent over the end of the tension wire and impacted into the proximal segment.

Alternatively, the fracture can initially be stabilized with two parallel small fragment screws or a partially threaded 6.5-mm cancellous screw placed down the shaft from the proximal piece. The wire loop is then placed to neutralize these constructs. The use of screws may offset some of the reported difficulties of the K wires backing out, causing discomfort and limited range of motion.

Some have advocated the use of a heavy nonabsorbable suture in place of wire to avoid the problem of wire breakage and pain on the subcutaneous border of the ulna. Even with these technique modifications, many patients will have hardware related issues that will require metal removal after fracture union.

Comminuted fractures (Fig. 1) and fractures involving the coronoid process or those that extend down the shaft of the ulna are not amenable to tension-band wiring. These fractures require interfragmentary reduction and neutralization with a plate in order to restore the anatomy and elbow stability. This plate, placed on the dorsal or dorsolateral surface of the ulna, functions as a neutralization device and a tension band. A 3.5-mm compression plate, one-third tubular plate, or pelvic reconstruction plate can be contoured to extend from the tip of the olecranon, across the fracture, and down the shaft of the ulna as needed. The 3.5-mm compression plate is bulky and can be more difficult to contour than the pelvic plate. A one-third tubular plate has a low profile but may not be strong enough to resist bending forces, especially in fractures that have no inherent stability from the bony reduction. Bone graft may be added to support a depressed articular segment, and lag screws can be placed from outside or through the plate to provide optimal fixation.

In highly comminuted fractures, particularly in the elderly, some have advocated olecranon excision and triceps reattachment as an alternative method of treatment. Poor bone quality or a highly comminuted fracture may make the fracture not amenable to reconstruction. The advantages of excision are that it is easy and rapid, eliminates the possibility of delayed union, nonunion, or posttraumatic arthritis; and allows early range of motion. The disadvantage of excision is said to be triceps weakness, elbow instability, and loss of motion. Rettig (6) found elbow motion to be equal after internal fixation or excision. Gartsman (7) found range of motion, elbow stability, and strength to be equal in patients who underwent open reduction compared to those who underwent excision. However, Gartsman's technique was not uniform and the elbow was immobilized in the postoperative period, delaying functional aftercare. Excision of the proximal ulna, though an option in difficult cases, cannot be advocated as the primary surgical treatment for this fracture.

III. FRACTURES OF THE PROXIMAL RADIUS

Fractures of the proximal radius are common and may represent 20% of all elbow trauma. While much has been written about their treatment, the definitive method remains controversial. With most intraarticular fractures, open reduction and rigid internal fixation is the key to good results. However, the proximal radius is an exception, as the exact mechanical role of the proximal radius is unclear. While the proximal radius provides some stability to valgus stress, the medial collateral ligament of the elbow is the primary stabilizer of the elbow (8–11). Acute excision of the radial head can lead to a loss of strength, valgus instability, and proximal migration of the radius with disruption of the wrist,

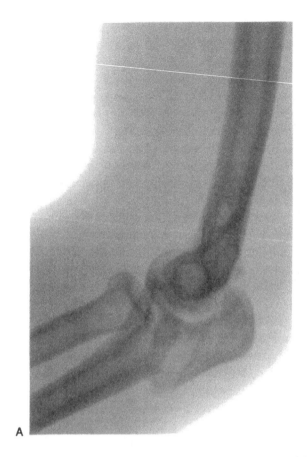

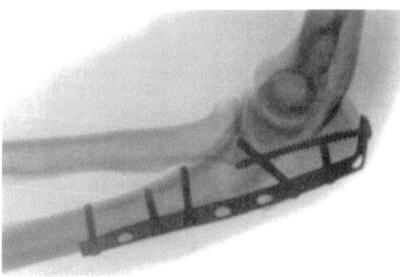

Figure 1 A. Displaced comminuted fracture of the olecranon. B. The fracture is stabilized by a tension band plating technique.

while late excision of the proximal radius does not appear to be fraught with these problems. In addition, reliably good implants for the fixation in this fracture are just being developed. This has led to a variety of treatment regimens for the radial head, with everything from long-term immobilization to aggressive open reduction and internal fixation being advocated.

Radial head fractures are usually the result of a fall on the outstretched hand. They may be associated with other injuries to the forearm and elbow, including the ulnar shaft, as is found in the Monteggia fracture.

An isolated fracture of the radial head usually causes pain on the lateral side of the elbow, which is aggravated by forearm rotation. Radial head fractures may be associated with a loss of full pronation and supination above that which may be expected from just pain and swelling. When a radial head fracture is suspected, the forearm and wrist must also be examined for pain and swelling. If wrist pain is present, radioulnar dissociation with injury to the interosseous ligament of the forearm should be suspected.

Routine anteroposterior (AP) and lateral radiographs of the elbow are essential for diagnosis. They may, however, not provide all information necessary. The radiocapitellar view can be helpful (12). This view is obtained by positioning the patient for a lateral x-ray but angling the beam 45 degrees toward the shoulder. If proximal radial migration is suspected, films of the wrist must be obtained to check the ulnar variance. When there is doubt, films of the contralateral side should be obtained for comparison.

The initial treatment of a radial head fracture should consist of splinting the patient for comfort. Aspirating the elbow joint through the radiocapitellar joint is useful not only to look for intraarticular hematoma but also to inject a local anesthetic for pain relief (13). A comfortable patient can be more thoroughly examined and the presence of a block to forearm rotation can be discovered. If there is a bony block to forearm or elbow motion as a result of a displaced radial head fracture, this is an indication for operative treatment.

There have been many classifications of radial head fractures. Most of these classifications have been based on radiographic findings, and the most commonly used has been that of Mason (14). None of the radiographic classifications takes into account the functional status of the proximal radioulnar joint. For that reason, I prefer to use the classification of Mason as modified by Hotchkiss. This classification is based on the patient's radiographic fracture pattern, physical signs, and associated injuries.

According to Hotchkiss (15) a type 1 fracture is nondisplaced or minimally displaced. Forearm rotation is limited only by pain and swelling, and intraarticular displacement is less than 2 mm. A type II fracture is displaced greater than 2 mm. Motion may be mechanically limited. The fracture is not severely comminuted and is amenable to internal fixation. Type 3 fractures are severely comminuted. They are not reconstructable and have a bony block to movement. They require radial head excision to regain motion. These fractures may involve an injury to the interosseous membrane and thus the wrist.

Nondisplaced or type 1 fractures can be treated nonoperatively. Most authors have reported that a brief period of immobilization followed by early functional rehabilitation produces good long-term results (16). Care must be taken in allowing early motion for fractures that involve a large majority of the articular surface, as these may displace. In the average patient, a period of immobilization of 1 to 2 weeks followed by active motion exercises will yield good results. Some loss of extension can be expected, but this does not occur in all fractures. Contracture, pain, and posttraumatic arthritis can occur despite what appears to be a well-aligned and minimally displaced fracture initially.

Treatment of type II fractures is more controversial. As noted earlier, Mason's classification is purely radiographic and did not take into account the functional status of the proximal radius. Examination of the elbow and radioulnar joints after the administration of local anesthesia can be very helpful in determining a treatment plan.

Type II fractures that do not involve a mechanical block to motion can be treated as type 1 fractures. If the patient has continued pain and stiffness after fracture union and an appropriate functional rehabilitation, a delayed radial head excision can be performed after any injury of the interosseous membrane has healed.

If the patient has a mechanical block to motion, the fracture should be treated operatively. Improvements in implant design have recently made this fracture more amenable to open reduction and internal fixation. The surgical approach to the radial head is through the lateral Kocher approach, exploiting the interval between the triceps and anconeus. Through a longitudinal capsulotomy, the fracture hematoma is debrided and adequate exposure is achieved. Care must be taken not to take down the annular ligament. If the annular ligament must be disrupted to gain appropriate exposure, it must be repaired prior to closure. Most often, the fracture will involve the anterolateral portion of the radial head. Care must be taken to avoid putting implants where they will impinge on either the proximal ulna or distal humerus. After anatomical reduction, fractures can be stabilized with K wires, minifragment 2.7- (Fig. 2) or 2.0-mm screws, or small buttress and blade plates. Simple fractures can be compressed with Herbert screws. Impaction of articular fragments can be elevated with bone grafting. As in type 1 fractures, late pain, loss of motion, and impairment can be treated with late radial head excision.

Type 3 injuries or comminuted fractures involving the entire radial head and neck are generally not reconstructable. If there is no injury to the interosseous membrane, early radial head excision can be successful. If, however, there is an interosseous membrane injury, early radial head excision will result in a proximal migration of the radius and disruption of the distal radioulnar joint. For this reason, early radial head excision should be accompanied by the implantation of a "spacer" to maintain the length of the radius and protect the interosseous ligament until it heals. Originally, radial head prostheses were developed from silicone. These implants have not been proven durable in the long term. Because

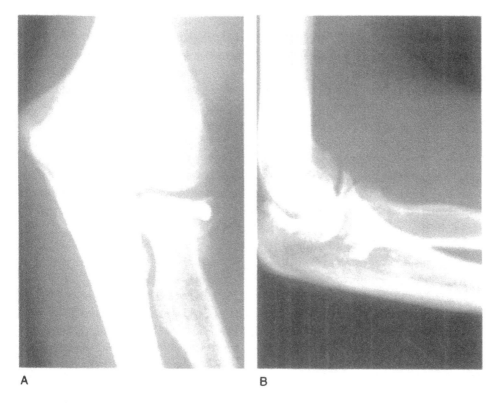

A   B

Figure 2   Anteroposterior (A) and lateral (B) films of a Mason type II fracture stabilized by open reduction and internal fixation through a Kocher approach.

of this, a wide variety of metallic implants are now available. These are modular and durable; they come in many sizes to more closely restore anatomical relationships. Some authors have reported the need to remove these prosthetic "spacers" after a period of time because of loosening. At that point, the interosseous ligament should have healed and late functional problems been avoided.

IV.   FRACTURES OF BOTH FOREARM BONES

There are many ways to fracture both bones of the forearm. The most common mechanism of injury is a direct blow. This may occur in a motor vehicle accident, fight, or fall from a height. Gunshot wounds can also cause a forearm fracture involving both bones and can result in neurovascular injury, a highly comminuted fracture, and extensive soft tissue injury.

Classifications of both-bone forearm fractures are usually descriptive. It is more useful to describe the bone involved, the segment of the bone involved, the degree of displacement, the presence or absence of bone loss and comminution, and whether the fracture is open or closed. Each of these factors has a prognostic implication as to the method of treatment and outcome of the fracture. The AO Comprehensive Classification of fractures has been adopted by many investigators and journals and is a useful way to compare like injuries. Disruption of the proximal or distal radioulnar joint is also important to note and will influence the method of treatment. The presence or absence of associated intraarticular fractures and whether the elbow, wrist, or radioulnar joints are involved is also important, so that treatment of other segments of the upper extremity may be coordinated.

In adults, nondisplaced fractures of the radius and ulna are rare. Fractures of both bones of the forearm are usually obvious clinically because the fractures are displaced. Symptoms include pain, deformity, and loss of function in the forearm and hand. Palpation of the forearm usually produces tenderness at the level of the fracture. Swelling is common.

The physical examination of the forearm should include a careful motor and sensory examination of all three major nerves. Radial, median, and ulnar nerve function should be documented. Neurological deficits, though not common, do occur. The presence or absence of pulses and their relationship to the contralateral extremity should be detailed. Both bone fractures of the forearm are a common cause of compartment syndrome. Tense swelling of the forearm may indicate the need for further investigation and possibly an urgent compartment release. The integrity of the skin should also be examined for signs of an open injury.

Standard radiographic evaluation of the forearm requires a minimum of two views. AP and lateral views are mandatory in all suspected forearm fractures. Oblique views of the elbow and of the wrist may be helpful. As always, it is imperative to include the joints above and below the suspected injury. Thus, in evaluating a suspected both-bones forearm fracture, it is important that both the wrist and the elbow be visualized. The presence or absence of joint subluxation or dislocation, especially with a one-bone forearm fracture, is important to note. A line drawn through the radial shaft, neck, and head should pass through the center of the capitellum on any projection taken. More advanced studies, such as computed tomography (CT) scans and magnetic resonance imaging (MRI) examinations, are usually not required.

Sarmiento and others (17,18) have shown that malunions as small as 10 degrees in any plane or in rotation can result in significant loss of pronation and supination and thus function of the forearm. For this reason, most forearm fractures in adults are treated with open anatomical reduction and rigid internal fixation (Fig. 3). This virtually guarantees maintenance of anatomical relationships and the ability to begin early functional rehabilitation. Nonoperative treatment is probably a more radical choice and is indicated only if there is a contraindication to surgery. Casts and cast braces (18) are useful only in the rare nondisplaced fracture. Even then, a long arm cast in full supination with the elbow flexed to 90 degrees is required.

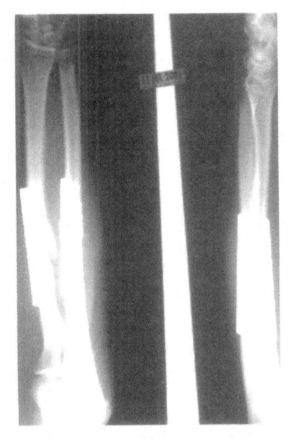

Figure 3 Final union films of a fracture of both bones of the forearm treated with plate fixation. The radial bow has been maintained.

Fractures of both bones of the forearm should be operated upon as soon as convenient (19). Early operative treatment permits decompression of the fracture hematoma, and reduction of the fracture fragments can minimize further soft tissue injury. In cases of poor soft tissue or in the multiply injured patient, surgery may be delayed as needed to allow either the patient's systemic problems or local soft tissue problems to resolve.

The majority of both-bones forearm fractures can be approached with the patient in the supine position. The hand table is commonly used, and many surgeons prefer to use an image intensifier during the procedure. A pneumatic tourniquet is helpful to increase visibility, but it must be let down prior to wound closure. Fixation with small-fragment 3.5-mm plates and screws has become the standard for these fractures. Though large-fragment 4.5-mm plates and screws have been shown to result in a similar rate of union, removal of these implants has a higher late refracture rate (19). In patients with small bones, 2.7-mm minifragment compression plates can be utilized. One-third tubular plates are not strong enough to resist bending forces and are associated with a higher degree of implant failure. In patients with severe soft tissue injury, burns, or bone loss, a provisional external fixator can allow restoration of alignment while waiting for soft tissue problems to resolve (20). If there is soft tissue loss, the external fixator can be maintained until definitive bone reconstruction is indicated.

The ulna lies in a subcutaneous position throughout the length of the forearm. The only significant structure that crosses the subcutaneous border of the ulna is the dorsal cutaneous branch of the ulnar nerve, which passes onto the dorsal surface of the flexor carpi ulnaris muscle 7 cm proximal to the ulnar styloid. Thus, approaches to the ulnar shaft involve an incision made over the subcutaneous border of the ulna, between the flexor and extensor masses. The plate can be applied to either the dorsal or volar surface of the bone, depending on the amount of stripping that has occurred or the preference of the surgeon. If it can be avoided, the plate should not be placed on the subcutaneous border of the ulna, as this may result in late irritation of the soft tissues and the need for subsequent plate removal.

There are two surgical approaches to the shaft of the radius: the volar approach of Henry and the dorsal approach of Thompson. The Henry approach is extensile, permitting easy extension of the exposure across the elbow or onto the hand. Any fracture of the radius can be fixed through the Henry approach, which is useful for creating forearm fasciotomies. This approach becomes more difficult proximally, with the presence of a number of neurovascular structures on the anterior aspect of the elbow. The dorsal approach is advantageous for the middle third of the radius. In this section, the radius is subcutaneous, and this approach provides easy access to the radial shaft. Though this approach allows the plate to be placed on the tensile surface of the bone, the dorsal approach is not extensile and thus cannot be used for complex injuries or forearm fasciotomies.

The forearm is a ring structure comprising two bones. Reduction of one bone will aid in bringing the other out to length. It is advisable to expose both fractures and provisionally fix the least comminuted fracture first. This facilitates reduction of the more comminuted side. Accuracy of the reduction can be assessed by evaluating the interdigitation of the fracture fragments and the contour of the cortex. After both fractures have been provisionally fixed, pronation and supination can be checked on the table and check x-rays obtained. If full motion is not present, the fracture must be taken down and reduced again.

A discussion of AO plating techniques is beyond the scope of this text. Interfragmentary compression should be utilized when possible (21). Transverse fractures should be stabilized with dynamic plate compression. Short oblique and spiral fractures can be provisionally fixed with lag screws and then neutralized with the plate. The management of comminuted fractures is more problematic. The surgeon should take great care to avoid stripping and preserve the soft tissue attachments to all of the comminuted fragments. Often, multiple fragments can be reduced using indirect techniques and then internally splinted by a bridging plate. This allows maintenance of fracture biology and provides both rotational and length stability. Segmental fractures can be treated with two plates if one plate is not long enough, but the plates should be placed at 90 degrees to each other if possible. Primary bone grafting of comminuted fractures was advocated by Anderson and produced results for these fractures similar to those obtained in closed noncomminuted fractures. With the use of more modern, biologically friendly plating techniques, the need for bone grafting in these high-energy injuries has not been demonstrated.

Care must be taken to avoid soft tissue stripping and manipulation of the radius and ulna along the interosseous membrane. If fractures are bone-grafted, the graft should not be placed in the area between the bones. Though synostosis of the radius and the ulna is a rare complication, it occurs more frequently in patients with comminuted fractures, crushing injuries to the upper extremity with a higher-grade soft tissue injury, or a concomitant head injury.

After surgery, the patient should be splinted until the wound is sealed. After suture removal, early motion can be started. Use of the arm is permitted for activities of daily living, with a weight-lifting restriction of 2 to 5 lb implemented. It is important to begin early finger, wrist, rotational, and elbow range of motion. These fractures usually heal in 3 to 4 months. Unlimited heavy physical activity should be restricted until solid remodeling has occurred, as documented by the radiographs.

V. GALEAZZI FRACTURES

Isolated, nondisplaced fractures of the radial shaft are rare in adults. Most injuries with sufficient energy to fracture the radius will also cause an injury to the ulna or the distal radioulnar joint. Any patient with an isolated radial shaft fracture should be suspected of having an additional injury. Truly isolated fractures may be treated nonoperatively, with most requiring a long arm cast. Frequent follow-up radiographs are necessary to detect late displacement. If displacement occurs, open reduction and internal fixation is essential to preventing loss of function.

More commonly, isolated fractures of the radial shaft at the junction of the middle and distal third is associated with an injury to the distal radioulnar joint. This fracture is commonly referred to as the Galeazzi fracture (Fig. 4). It has also been called a reverse Monteggia fracture, a Piedmont fracture, and a "fracture of necessity" (22,23). The distinguishing feature of this injury is a subluxation or dislocation of the distal radioulnar joint.

This injury is rare, with an incidence of only 3 to 6% of all forearm fractures. The hallmark of this injury is a clinically apparent radial shaft fracture with the addition of swelling and pain at the distal radioulnar joint. Radiographically, disruption of the distal radioulnar joint is suggested by a fracture of the ulnar

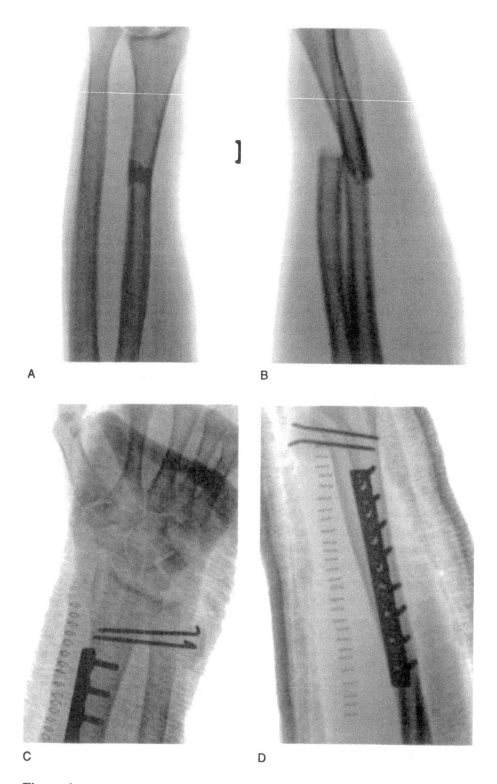

Figure 4 Anteroposterior (A) and lateral (B) films of a Galeazzi fracture. Postoperatively (C and D) the radius has been plated out to length and the radioulnar joint reduced and held with two K wires.

styloid at its base, widening of the distal radioulnar joint space on the AP radiograph, dislocation of the radius relative to the ulna on the lateral radiograph, and shortening of the radius greater than 5 mm (24).

It is generally recognized that a Galeazzi fracture is best treated operatively (22,23). Difficulties with nonoperative treatment were confirmed by Hughston in 1957. He identified unsatisfactory results in 35 of the 38 cases treated by closed reduction in his series.

These fractures of the distal third of the radius are best approached by the volar Henry exposure (25). The fracture of the radial shaft is treated by standard AO techniques, and the plate is placed on the volar surface of the radius. At this point, standard AP and lateral radiographs are obtained. If the distal radioulnar joint has been reduced, stability is assessed. This can be done by palpating the distal ulna relative to the radius and examining the distal radioulnar joint in pronation. If the distal radioulnar joint is stable throughout the range of motion, there is no need for postoperative immobilization, and early functional rehabilitation can begin.

If reduction of the distal radioulnar joint is present in supination but not in pronation, stability must be provided. If there is an associated fracture of the ulnar styloid, this can be operatively repaired to provide stability. Alternatively, two 2.0-mm K wires can be placed between radius and ulna just proximal to the distal radioulnar joint. These wires are placed with the forearm held in full supination to guarantee a stable reduction of the distal radioulnar joint. The arm is immobilized in full supination, and the elbow can begin early range of motion in flexion and extension. The wires are maintained for 3 to 4 weeks and can be removed in the clinic. If the distal radioulnar joint cannot be reduced in this injury, soft tissue interposition in the joint should be suspected (26,27). The joint should be exposed and explored from the dorsal approach. The most common soft tissue interposed is the extensor carpi ulnaris tendon.

VI. ISOLATED ULNAR FRACTURES

Isolated fractures of the ulnar shaft not associated with injury to the proximal radioulnar joint are common. These injuries are often caused by a direct blow to ulnar shaft and are often called *nightstick fractures*, after patients having been injured while assuming a defensive position. These fractures are often nondisplaced or minimally displaced.

Many forms of treatment for nondisplaced isolated ulnar shaft fractures have been suggested. Some authors have advocated casual treatment with an Ace wrap (28), while others have advocated long arm casts or operative treatment. Sarmiento and others as well as Zych (29) have pointed out that isolated nondisplaced fractures of the ulnar shaft can be treated in a functional brace. These fractures require angulation of less than 10 degrees and a reliable patient. Any fracture with a vascular or neurological deficit should be treated operatively.

Fractures that are angulated more than 10 degrees in any plane or displaced more than 50% of the diameter of the diaphysis have been classified as displaced by Dymond (30). He felt that these fractures were more unpredictable and should be approached with caution. They are more often associated with subtle instability of the proximal radioulnar joint, are prone to further angulation, and can shorten. For this reason, displaced isolated fractures of the ulnar shaft should probably be treated with initial open reduction and internal fixation.

VII. MONTEGGIA FRACTURES

Monteggia originally described this injury as a fracture of the proximal third of ulna with associated anterior dislocation of the radial epiphysis. Bado (31) expanded the term *Monteggia lesion* to include any fracture of the proximal third of the ulna with associated radioulnar pathology.

This fracture is characterized by swelling about the elbow and deformity as well as bony crepitus and pain at the fracture site. Often, one can palpate the dislocated radial head. A thorough neurological and vascular examination is necessary, because injury to the radial nerve as it comes around the radial neck is not uncommon.

True AP and lateral x-rays of the elbow must be obtained. The forearm and wrist joint must also be visualized. Although the fracture of the ulna is usually obvious, the dislocation of the radial head can be subtle. A line drawn through the radial tuberosity, radial neck, and radial head should always pass through the center of the capitellum. This is a constant on all x-ray views and can be useful in diagnosing subtle instabilities.

Bado described four distinct variations of this fracture. A type 1 injury is a fracture of the ulnar diaphysis at any level with anterior angulation at the fracture site and associated anterior dislocation of the radial head. This is considered to be the most common type of lesion. A type II injury consists of a fracture of the ulnar diaphysis with posterior angulation of the fracture site and a posterolateral dislocation of the radial head. A type 3 lesion is a fracture of the ulnar metaphysis with a lateral or anterolateral dislocation of the radial head. A type 4 lesion is a fracture of the proximal third of the radius and ulna the same level with anterior dislocation of the radial head.

While closed treatment is an acceptable option in some pediatric patients, the adult patient should be treated with open reduction and internal fixation (Fig. 5). The ulnar shaft must be anatomically reduced and securely fixed in order to accurately position the radial head. Restoration of the length of the ulna restores the length of the forearm. This usually results in a closed reduction of the proximal radioulnar joint.

Once an anatomical reconstruction of the ulnar shaft is been accomplished, stability of the proximal radioulnar joint must be assessed. Stability of the radial head with range of motion—in both flexion/extension and pronation/supination—must be achieved. Instability of the proximal radius may indicate an inadequate reduction of the ulna. In cases of bone loss or open fractures, it can be difficult to determine the appropriate length of the bone.

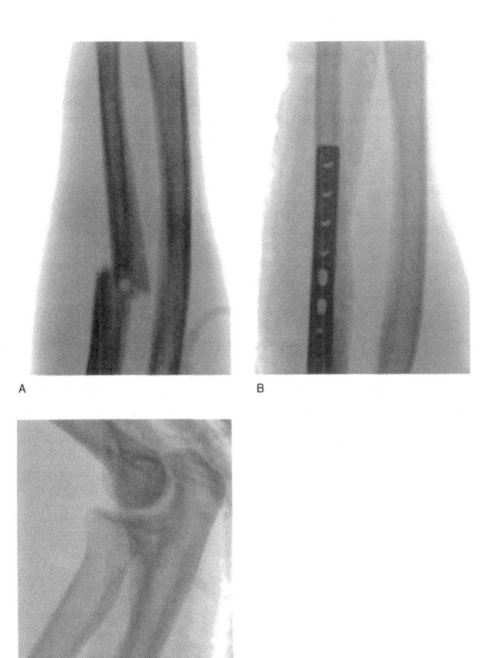

Figure 5 A Monteggia fracture (A). Postoperatively (B and C) the ulna has been anatomically reduced, which results in the closed anatomical restoration of the proximal radioulnar joint.

If the radial head cannot be relocated despite an anatomical reduction of the ulna, the proximal radioulnar joint must be opened and reduced directly. Injuries to the annular ligament must be repaired directly. In associated fractures of the radial head, removal of interposed bone fragments may result in an adequate reduction.

REFERENCES

1. E Schemitsch, R Richards. The effect of malunion on functional outcome after plate fixation of fractures of both bones of the forearm in adults. J Bone Joint Surg Am 74A:1068–1078, 1992.

2. R Hotchkiss, K An, D Sowa, S Basta, A Weiland. An anatomic and mechanical study of the interosseous membrane of the forearm: Pathomechanics of proximal migration of the radius. J Hand Surg [Am] 14A:256–261, 1989.

3. C Colton. Fractures of the olecranon in adults: Classification and management. Injury 5:121–129, 1973–1974.

4. M Muller, M Allgower, R Schneider, H Willenegger. Manual of Internal Fixation, 2nd ed. Berlin: Springer-Verlag, 1979.

5. D Murphy, W Greene, T Dameron. Displaced olecranon fractures in adults: Clinical evaluation. Clin Orthop 224:215–223, 1987.

6. A Rettig, T Waugh, P Evanski. Fracture of the olecranon: A problem of management. J Trauma 19:23–28, 1979.

7. G Gartsman, T Sculco, J Otis. Operative treatment of olecranon fractures—Excision or open reduction with internal fixation. J Bone Joint Surg Am 63A:718–721, 1981.

8. BF Morrey, KN An. Articular and ligamentous contributions to the stability of the elbow joint. Am J Sports Med 11:315–319, 1983.

9. BF Morrey, KN An, TJ Stormont. Force transmission through the radial head. J Bone Joint Surg Am 70: 250–256, 1988.

10. BF Morrey, EY Chao, FC Hui. Biomechanical study of the elbow following excision of the radial head. J Bone Joint Surg Am 61:63–68, 1979.

11. BF Morrey, S Tanaka, KN An. Valgus stability of the elbow. A definition of primary and secondary constraints. Clin Orthop 187–195, 1991.

12. N Greenspan, A Norman. The radial head capitellar view: Useful technique in elbow trauma. Am J Roentgenol 8:1186–1190, 1982.

13. T Quigly. Aspiration of the elbow joint in treatment of fractures of the head and neck of the radius. N Engl J Med 240:915–916, 1949.

14. M Mason. Some observations on fractures of the head of the radius with a review of one hundred cases. Br J Surg 42:123–132, 1954.

15. R Hotchkiss. Fractures and dislocations of the elbow. In: Heckman J, ed. Rockwood and Green's Fractures in Adults. Philadelphia: Lippincott-Raven, 1996, pp 929–1024.

16. H McLaughlin. Trauma. Philadelphia: Saunders, 1959.

17. RR Tarr, AI Garfinkel, A Sarmiento. The effects of angular and rotational deformities of both bones of the forearm. An in vitro study. J Bone Joint Surg Am 66: 65–70, 1984.

18. A Sarmiento, JS Cooper, WF Sinclair. Forearm fractures. Early functional bracing—A preliminary report. J Bone Joint Surg Am 57:297–304, 1975.

19. MW Chapman, JE Gordon, AG Zissimos. Compression-plate fixation of acute fractures of the diaphyses of the radius and ulna. J Bone Joint Surg Am 71:159–169, 1989.

20. T Grace, W Eversman. The management of segmental bone loss associated with forearm fractures. J Bone Joint Surg Am 58A:283–284, 1976.

21. LD Anderson, D Sisk, RE Tooms, WI Park, III. Compression-plate fixation in acute diaphyseal fractures of the radius and ulna. J Bone Joint Surg Am 57(3):287, 1975.

22. J Hughston. Fracture of the distal radius shaft: Mistakes in management. J Bone Joint Surg Am 39A:249–264, 1957.

23. M Stewart. Discussion of paper. J Bone Joint Surg Am 39A:264, 1957.

24. JD Bruckner, DM Lichtman, AH Alexander. Complex dislocations of the distal radioulnar joint. Recognition and management. Clin Orthop 275:90–103, 1992.

25. W Henry. Extensile exposures, 2nd ed. New York: Churchill Livingstone, 1973, p 100.

26. AH Alexander, DM Lichtman. Irreducible distal radioulnar joint occurring in a Galeazzi fracture—Case report. J Hand Surg [Am] 6:258–261, 1981.

27. A Biyani, S Bhan. Dual extensor tendon entrapment in Galeazzi fracture-dislocation: A case report. J Trauma 29:1295–1297, 1989.

28. M Hoffer, W Schobert. The failure of casual treatment for nondisplaced ulna shaft fractures. J Trauma 24:771–773, 1984.

29. G Zych, L Latta, J Zagorski. Treatment of isolated ulnar shaft fractures with prefabricated functional fracture braces. Clin Orthop 219:194–200, 1987.

30. I Dymond. The treatment of isolated fractures of the distal ulna. J Bone Joint Surg Br 66B:408–410, 1984.

31. JL Bado. The Monteggia lesion. Clin Orthop 50:71–86, 1967.

4

Intraarticular Fractures of the Distal Humerus

Rob Dawson, Mark E. Baratz, and William Greer
Allegheny General Hospital, Pittsburgh, Pennsylvania, U.S.A.

Intraarticular fractures of the distal humerus challenge both surgeon and patient. The patient, having sudden and significant impairment of a limb, expects guidance regarding treatment and a reliable prediction regarding the ultimate functioning of the affected arm. The surgeon's ability to provide excellent care and an accurate prognosis depends on his or her skill in assessing the injury, performing the surgery, and managing the rehabilitation.

I. EVALUATION

The key to initiating care and formulating a prognosis is developing an accurate evaluation of the energy of the injury, the condition of the soft tissues, and the fracture pattern.

Fractures of the distal humerus result from a wide variety of injuries. The specifics of the accident help to determine the energy of the injury and are essential in recommending appropriate treatment. Rehabilitation following a crush injury will be much different from that needed to treat a fall on an outstretched arm. Assessment of the condition of the soft tissues must include a careful inspection to identify puncture wounds or abrasions that might be indicative of an open fracture. Evaluation of the soft tissues involves assessment of limb vascularity and nerve function, particularly the ulnar nerve, which is properly assessed via two-point discrimination in the ring and small fingers. Intrinsic muscle function is assessed by measuring the strength of the abducted index finger, palpating the first dorsal interosseous muscle, and asking the patient to cross the middle finger over the index finger (Fig. 1A to C).

A. Imaging

Imaging is the most important component of preoperative planning and postoperative prognosis. It can be accomplished with plain radiographs, tomography, or computerized tomography (CT) scans. The traction radiograph, taken in the operating room, is usually adequate to assess the quality of the condyles and the extent of intraarticular comminution (Fig. 2A and B); it is also cost-effective.

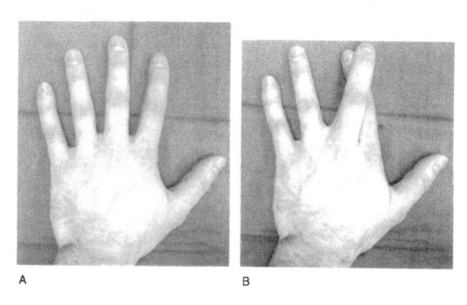

A   B

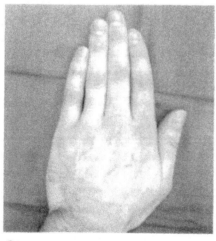

C

Figure 1   Ulnar nerve motor function is assessed by (A) finger abduction, (B) adduction, and (C) crossing the middle finger over the index finger.

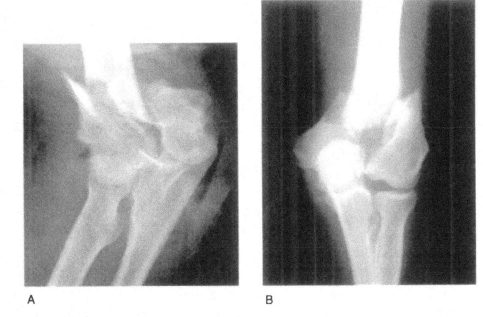

A   B

Figure 2   A. AP Radiograph of a comminuted distal humerus fracture. B. AP Traction
radiograph of same fracture more clearly demonstrating fracture pattern.

B. Fracture Classification

Many classification systems have been described for fractures of the distal humerus. Morrey et al. divided these fractures into three main groups: extraarticular, intraarticular, and extracapsular (1). The Arbeitsgemeinschaft für Osteosynthe-
sefragen/Association for the Study of Internal Fixation (AO/ASIF) system
describes three types of fractures: type A, extraarticular fractures; type B, fractures of part of the articular surface in which a portion remains attached proximally; and type C, where there is no connection with the supporting osseous
structures. The AO/ASIF classification is further broken down into 27 subgroups
based on location and orientation of the major fracture lines and the degree of
metaphyseal and articular comminution (2). Intraarticular fractures are further
subdivided into single-column fractures, bicolumn fractures, capitellar fractures,
and trochlear fractures. The Jupiter and Mehne classification is used in this chapter (3) (Table 1).

II. TREATMENT

A. Surgical Consent

A preview of the course of treatment, including a discussion of the potential
risks, not only helps the patient put his injury into perspective but serves as an
essential hedge against medicolegal risk. Potential negative outcomes of surgery
include nerve or vessel injury, infection, reflex sympathetic dystrophy, hardware

Table 1   Classification of Distal Humeral Fractures

I.   Intrarticular fractures
    A.   Single-column fractures
        1.   Medial
            a.   High
            b.   Low
        2.   Lateral
            a.   High
            b.   Low
        3.   Divergent
    B.   Bicolumn fractures
        1.   T pattern
            a.   High
            b.   Low
        2.   Y pattern
        3.   H pattern
        4.   Lambda pattern
            a.   Medial
            b.   Lateral
        5.   Multiplane pattern
    C.   Capitellar fractures
    D.   Trochlear fractures
II.   Extraarticular intracapsular fractures
    A.   Transcolumn fractures
        1.   High
            a.   Extension
            b.   Flexion
            c.   Abduction
            d.   Adduction
        2.   Low
            a.   Extension
            b.   Flexion
III.   Extracapsular fractures
    A.   Medial epicondyle
    B.   Lateral epicondyle

Source: Ref. 39.

failure, nonunion, malunion, elbow instability, elbow stiffness, and posttraumatic arthritis. Additional surgery may also be required.

B. Equipment

The "distal humerus tool kit" includes a large-tenaculum from the large fragment Synthes (Paoli, PA) set, 0.062 and 0.045 wires, a wire driver, the small-fragment Synthes set, and 3.5-mm reconstruction plates. Acumed has recently introduced a set of low-profile plates that are useful for T-condylar distal humeral fractures, particularly when the horizontal limb of the T is close to the articular surface (Fig. 3).

C. Anesthesia and Positioning

Most intraarticular distal humeral fractures are addressed through a posterior approach with the patient in a lateral position; it is useful here to support the brachium with a tibial leg holder that is mounted to the operating table (Fig. 4). We have successfully treated capitellar fractures through a lateral approach with the patient in the supine position.

D. Surgical Approaches

1. Posterior Approach

The incision for the posterior approach runs just medial to the tip of the olecranon. The ulnar nerve is identified as it passes through the cubital tunnel (Fig. 5A); it is mobilized so that it lies loosely in the subcutaneous tissues of the medial skin flap (Fig. 5B).

Exposure of the distal humerus can be accomplished in four ways: olecranon osteotomy, triceps retraction, a triceps "sparing," and triceps splitting. The olecranon osteotomy provides an exceptional view of the anterior and posterior aspects of the articular surface; its disadvantages are the risk of nonunion and prominent hardware. The olecranon osteotomy is performed at a level in the olecranon fossa where there is frequently an absence of cartilage (Fig. 6A and B). This bare area in articular cartilage can be localized by making a small opening in the joint capsule. Experience with olecranon osteotomy has shown a 30% incidence of nonunion with a transverse osteotomy (4). The recommended technique is to create a chevron osteotomy with a small oscillating saw. The cut is stopped just short of the subchondral bone and is completed by "cracking" the subchondral bone and cartilage with an osteotome. This creates an irregular spike that facilitates reduction and fixation of the fragments at the end of the procedure.

Baratz and Shanahan studied the morphology of the proximal ulna and identified several factors that have bearing on fixation of an olecranon osteotomy (5). The medullary canal of the proximal ulna is approximately 9 mm in diameter just distal to the coronoid process. Between 40 and 65 mm from the tip of the olecranon, the medullary canal narrows to 5.5 mm (Fig. 7). This is important if screw fixation is chosen to repair the osteotomized olecranon: a large-diameter screw may gain excellent purchase once it reaches a point 65 mm from the tip of the olecranon; however, if the cortical bone is dense, the screw may not advance, thereby limiting compression of the repaired olecranon osteotomy. Using a chevron osteotomy and screw fixation, Jones et al. had a 32% overall complication rate, 15% of which was due to nonunion when the osteotomy was fixed with a screw of 70 mm or less (6). As a result, they recommended chevron osteotomy

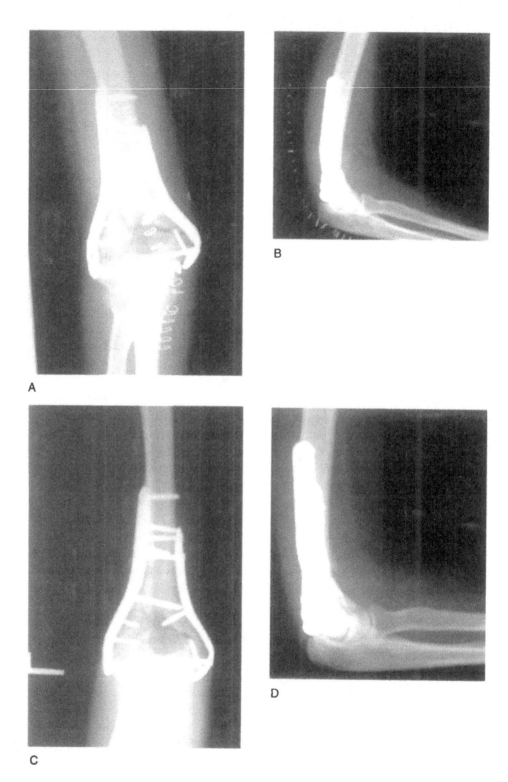

Figure 3 A-D. Patient who had the Acumed low-profile contoured plates implanted for a comminuted distal humerus fracture.

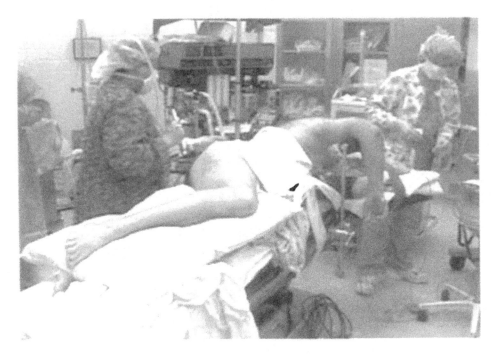

Figure 4   Placement of patient in the lateral position using tibial post.

with a screw that was 70 mm in length or longer with or without tension-band wiring. Our experience suggests tension-band wiring is best for fixing an olecranon osteotomy. Jupiter et al. have reported excellent success with a double-wiring technique (7) (Fig. 8). When an olecranon osteotomy is decided on, the fixation should be secure, so that no motion is visible at the osteotomy site when the elbow is taken through the full range of motion.

Retraction of the triceps is a technique used to expose the distal humerus in fractures where the fragments can easily be seen and reduced working medial or lateral to the triceps. The disadvantages to this approach are limited visibility of the articular surface and the need for indirect reduction.

The triceps-sparing approach has the advantages of good view and low morbidity; it is, however, impossible to see the anterior aspect of the joint unless the collateral ligaments are released. A long sheet of the triceps is reflected off the olecranon working from medial to lateral (Fig. 9A and B). Retracting the triceps laterally provides an excellent view of the posterior aspects of the humerus and the articular surface. The triceps-sparing approach does not allow good visibility if the fracture extends proximally. This is particularly true in individuals who have a large triceps muscle. Divelbiss et al. found that the triceps-sparing approach provided adequate exposure and motion equivalent to that of reported results for the olecranon osteotomy; they reported two cases of transient radial nerve palsy when a metal retractor was used to retract the triceps (8). Their experience suggests that the triceps is best retracted with the hand.

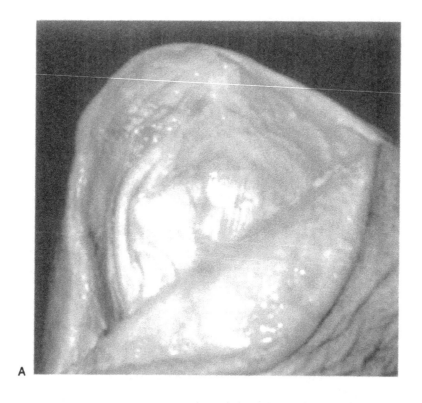

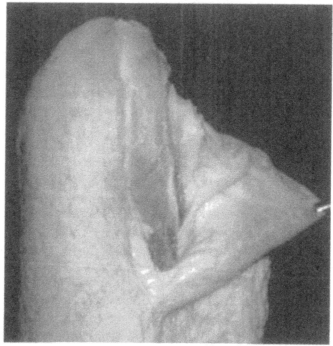

Figure 5 A. The ulnar nerve is identified in the cubital tunnel using the posterior approach to the elbow. B. The ulnar nerve is mobilized and should be protected throughout the surgery.

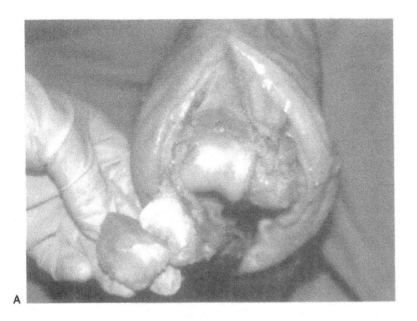

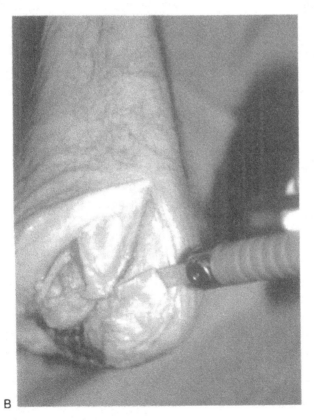

Figure 6 A. An olecranon osteotomy demonstrating the absence of articular cartilage at the osteotomy site. B. An oscillating saw is used when making the olecranon osteotomy. A chevron-type osteotomy is preferred and demonstrated.

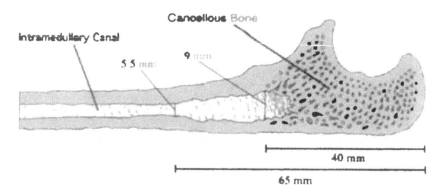

Figure 7 A schematic demonstrating the size of the ulnar medullary canal. (From Ref. 5.)

The triceps-splitting approach can be extended to expose the distal humerus: the triceps is split through its central portion and the insertion peeled off the tip of the olecranon. Balk and Ziran reported a modification of this technique, where the collateral ligaments were released medially and laterally to permit an unobstructed view of articular surface: in a series including 14 patients, they reported superior exposure and a 107-degree arc of elbow motion; three of the 14 patients had transient radial nerve palsies and two patients had asymptomatic valgus instability (9).

Anatomy Relevant to Fracture Fixation. The anatomy of the distal humerus is complex. Its accurate reconstruction requires a precise mental picture of normal anatomy. Optimal stabilization of fractures is accomplished by understanding optimal points of fixation.

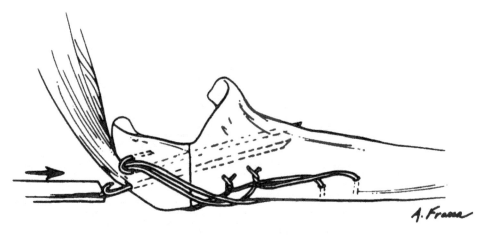

Figure 8 Double tension-band fixation of the olecranon. (From Ref. 7.)

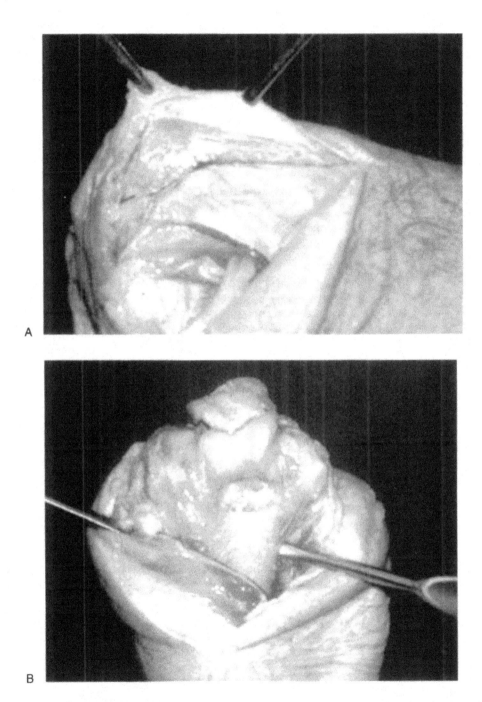

Figure 9 A-B. The triceps-sparring approach can allow for excellent visualization of the distal humerus.

The shaft of the humerus flattens as it nears the elbow and gives rise to two columns: lateral and medial. As the medial and lateral columns diverge distally around the olecranon fossa, they form a triangle, with the trochlea and capitellum combining to form the base. Recreation of this triangle is essential to accurate reconstruction of distal humeral fractures.

The distal humerus lies in 5 degrees of valgus and 30 degrees of flexion (Fig. 10A and B). Failure to restore valgus reflects malreduction of either the medial or lateral column. Failure to restore flexion will compromise the elbow's normal flexion-extension arc.

The medial aspect of the distal humerus has a complex contour that limits options for plate fixation. Precontoured plates may help alleviate some of the problems with plate fixation on the medial side.

There is a bare spot on the posterior aspect of the lateral condyle. This is an excellent location to place a plate for fixation of the lateral condyle or to place malleolar screws to secure fractures of the capitellum. There are anterior and posterior sulci on the anterior and posterior aspects of the lateral condyle at the proximal margins of the capitellum (Fig. 11A and B). A plate placed too far distally on the posterior aspect of the humerus will impinge against the radial head, blocking extension; a screw placed into the anterior sulcus of the capitel-

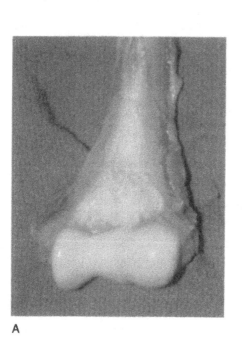
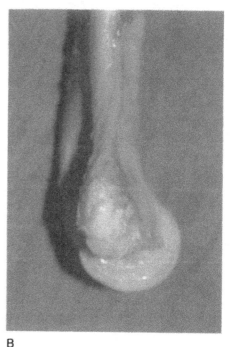

A   B

Figure 10   A-B. AP and lateral views of gross distal humerus specimens showing the complex contour of the bone.

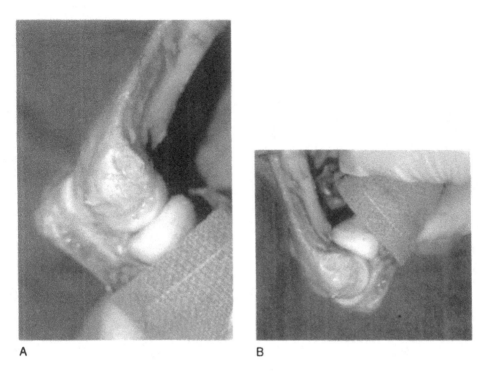

A   B

Figure 11   A-B. Gross specimens showing the anterior and posterior radial sulci. Note that placement of a plate too far anteriorly or posteriorly could cause impingement on the radial head.

lum will block flexion. The posterior aspect of the olecranon fossa creates a problem and a solution in the fixation of distal humerus fractures. Hardware cannot protrude into the fossa without blocking extension. However, the olecranon fossa is surrounded by strong cortical bone; screws placed into this bone but not into the olecranon fossa will provide an excellent purchase (Fig. 12A and B).

III. Capitellar Fractures

Fractures of the capitellum have an estimated incidence of 0.5 to 1.0% of all elbow fractures (10,11). Although Hahn described the first case in 1853, Kocher is credited with its description. Fractures of the capitellum are typically the result of shearing force delivered through the radial head, presumably during a fall with a partially flexed elbow. Bohler thought the fracture occurred when hyperextension of the elbow combined with a valgus stress; he also thought the fracture was frequently accompanied by a tear of the medial collateral ligament (12). In our experience, symptomatic medial collateral injuries are uncommon in patients with capitellar fractures.

There are two types of capitellar fractures. Type I, or Hahn-Steinthal fractures, involve a large portion of the capitellum and sometimes part of the trochlea

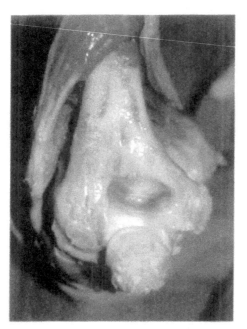 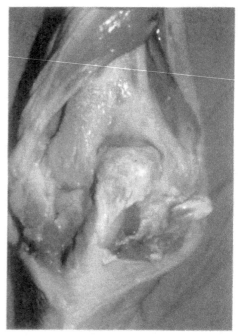

A   B

Figure 12   A. Gross specimen with the forearm extended shows the olecranon fossa.
B. Gross specimen with the forearm flexed demonstrates the articulation of the distal
humerus with the proximal ulna posteriorly.

(13–17). Type II, also known as Kocher-Lorenz fractures, involves articular cartilage with minimal subchondral bone. Capitellar fractures are diagnosed by routine radiographs and physical examination; there is often a mechanical block
to flexion with type I fractures and a block to extension with type II fractures. The
fracture may be difficult to visualize on anteroposterior (AP) radiographs but is
usually apparent on a lateral projection of the elbow. It typically displaces anteriorly and superiorly and is therefore easily seen in the area of the olecranon fossa.

Treatment of capitellar fractures is controversial. Some authors advocate
nonoperative treatment (14,15,18). Others recommend open reduction with internal fixation (16,17,19–21). Still others suggest excision of the fragment (14,21,
22). Nonoperative treatment is reserved for nondisplaced fractures. The elbow is
splinted for a short period, which is followed by protected motion. Although
some authors have advocated closed reduction of displaced fractures, the lack of
soft tissue attachment to the fragment makes a closed reduction difficult if not
impossible (21).

Operative intervention involves open reduction with internal fixation or
fragment excision. These fractures are typically treated by using a standard posterolateral (Kocher) approach to the elbow, whether the plan is excision or reduction with fixation. Once the fracture is visualized, care should be taken to pre-

serve any soft tissue attachments that remain; if reduction is planned, then adequate visualization is essential and the reduction must be perfect. It is also essential to assess the amount of subchondral bone present. Excision is the preferred treatment when there is little subchondral bone, the fragment is extensively comminuted, or perfect reduction cannot be achieved (14,21,22). Fixation of the capitellar fragment has been attempted with a number of devices, including the Herbert screw (23), Kirschner wires (24), and screws (16,17,19,21,25).

Screw fixation is usually accomplished by inserting a partially threaded screw from posterior to anterior as a lag screw. The screw can also be placed from anterior to posterior. If the fracture pattern makes this technique necessary, it is essential to countersink the head of the screw. Collert (19) reported on 20 patients treated with screw fixation; 7 had excellent results. Herbert screws have been reported in two small series with good results (23,26). The advantage of using a Herbert screw is that the screw head is small and can easily be countersunk beneath articular cartilage.

Advocates of fragment excision cite results superior to those in patients treated by other means. Alvarez reported on 10 patients treated in this fashion: 9 had good to excellent elbow motion, 3 reported only minimal pain, and 6 reported no pain; there were no reports of elbow instability or cubitus valgus (22).

Trochlear fractures in isolation are exceedingly rare even when compared to the number of capitellar fractures. The anatomy of the trochlea is such that it is not subject to the same shearing and compressive force as the capitellum. It has been noted that the shearing forces required to cause a trochlear fracture are achieved with an elbow dislocation (24).

If they are nondisplaced, fractures of the trochlea can be managed with 3 weeks of immobilization followed by mobilization. If the fragment is displaced, it is essential to open the joint and fix the fracture (26,27).

IV. BICONDYLAR FRACTURES

The incidence of bicondylar fractures is between 5 and 60% of all distal humeral fractures (28). These fractures have been divided into six different types by Mehne and Matta (29), based on the orientation of fracture fragments. Bicondylar fractures are often the result of a fall on the olecranon with the elbow flexed to greater than 90 degrees.

The Mehta classification addresses the characteristics of the fracture with the goal of assisting in preoperative planning. The different classes are as follows:

1. High T fracture—A transverse fracture that goes through the superior portion of the olecranon fossa or proximal to it (Fig. 13).
2. Low T fracture—A transverse fracture that passes through or distal to the olecranon fossa (Fig. 14).
3. Y fracture—Oblique fractures cross both medial and lateral column, join in the olecranon fossa, and extend vertically into the joint, splitting the trochlea (Fig. 15).

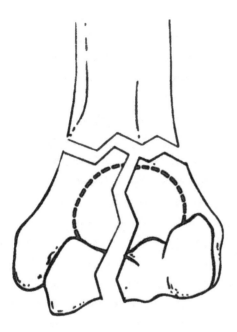

Figure 13   Schematic diagram of a high-T fracture. (From Ref. 39.)

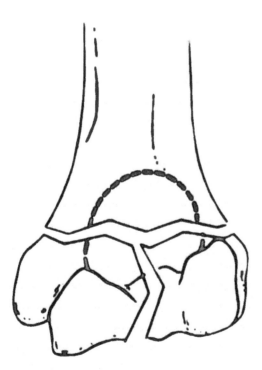

Figure 14   Schematic diagram of a low-T bicolumn fracture. (From Ref. 39.)

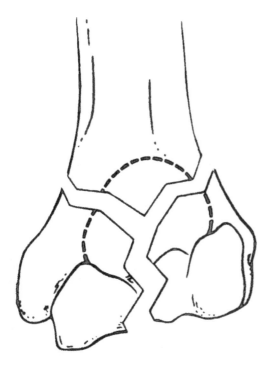

Figure 15 Schematic diagram of a Y bicolumn fracture. (From Ref. 39.)

4. H fracture—The medial column has a fracture proximal and distal to the medial epicondyle, and the lateral column is fractured in a T or Y pattern. The trochlea is a free fragment and may be further comminuted. In addition, the trochlea is at increased risk for avascular necrosis (Fig. 16).

5. Medial lambda fracture—The most proximal fracture line exits medially with the lateral fracture line distal to the lateral epicondyle, leaving a small zone for internal fixation on the lateral side (Fig. 17).

6. Lateral lambda fracture—The pattern is similar to that of an H fracture, but the lateral column is not involved (Fig. 18).

In addition to the above, there can always be a shearing force to the distal humerus, which occurs with these injuries or alone and results in a fracture pattern in the coronal plane, as described by Jupiter et al. (30).

V. FRACTURE REDUCTION AND FIXATION

The mainstay of treatment is open reduction with rigid internal fixation. However, there is some role for total elbow arthroplasty in the elderly with severe osteopenia. Until the early 1970s, most surgeons believed that the treatment of choice was nonoperative, because of unpredictable results with operative inter-

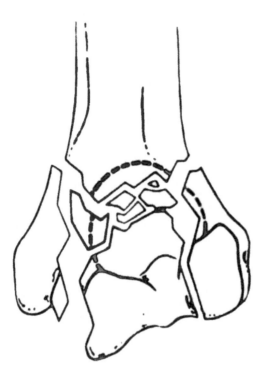

Figure 16   Schematic diagram of an H fracture. (From Ref. 39.)

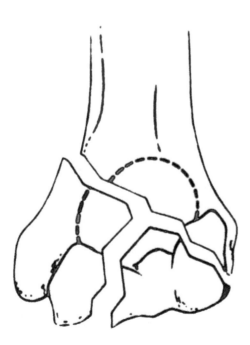

Figure 17   Schematic diagram of a medial lamda fracture. (From Ref. 39.)

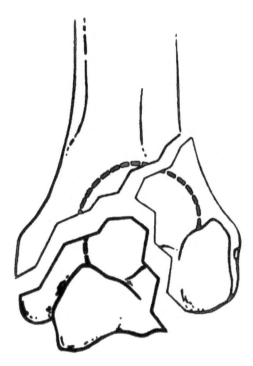

Figure 18 Schematic diagram of a lateral lambda fracture. (From Ref. 39.)

vention (13,31). Since that time, most authors have demonstrated favorable results with operative intervention.

A. Open Reduction and Internal Fixation

Fixation of distal humeral fractures has been a subject of research for a number of years. In 1993, Helfet recommended the use of a posterolateral dynamic compression plate (DCP) plate with a medial one-third tubular plate (32). Subsequently, Jacobson et al. recommended plate fixation with a posterior lateral DCP and a medial reconstruction plate (33). O'Driscoll has designed posterior, medial and lateral plates contoured to fit the bone.

There are usually three main parts to a bicondylar fracture of the distal humerus. Reduction and fixation of distal humeral fractures begins, in most cases, with reduction of the articular surface. When the articular surface is comminuted, the authors favor a "best fit" method of reduction in which the surgeon tries to find that portion of the humerus that best interdigitates with the distal fracture fragment and to build the fracture from there. This can be assisted with provisional pin fixation using 0.62 pins (Fig. 19). Once provisional fixation of a portion or an entire segment of a column has been accomplished, the fracture is stabilized with screws and plates. When the distal humerus is reconstructed, there may be discontinuity either within the metaphysis or within the cortex. If there

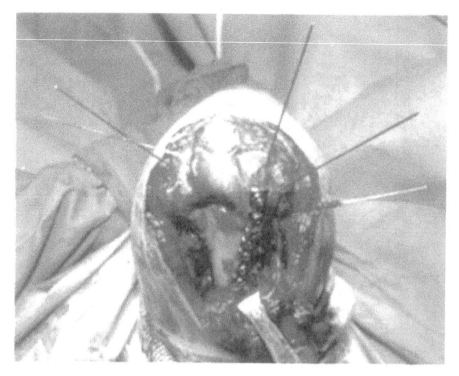

Figure 19   Intraoperative photograph of provisional fixation of a distal humerus fracture using kirschner wires.

is a defect in the construct, two types of bone graft can be used: structural graft or filler graft. Structural graft is used for cortical discontinuity. We recommend filling the defect with a press-fit portion of iliac crest bone graft. When there is cortical continuity with a metaphyseal defect, the defect can be filled with cancellous bone. Once fixation is accomplished, intraoperative radiographs are obtained. The triceps must be reconstructed by fixing the olecranon osteotomy or by repairing the sleeve of soft tissue back to bone. When the triceps mechanism has been reestablished, the elbow is placed through a range of motion to ensure there is no block to either flexion or extension.

B.   Total Elbow Arthroplasty

In general, total elbow arthroplasty in the setting of acute trauma is reserved for the elderly patient with a severely comminuted fracture (Figs. 20 to 22). The osteopenia in these patients makes open reduction with internal fixation very difficult. There is little in the literature about this option. The largest series, that of Cobb and Morrey, had 20 patients and 21 elbows treated acutely with total elbow replacements for comminuted distal humeral fractures (34). Using the Mayo elbow performance score, 15 patients in the study had excellent results and 5 good results. The mean age of patients in the study was 72 at the time of

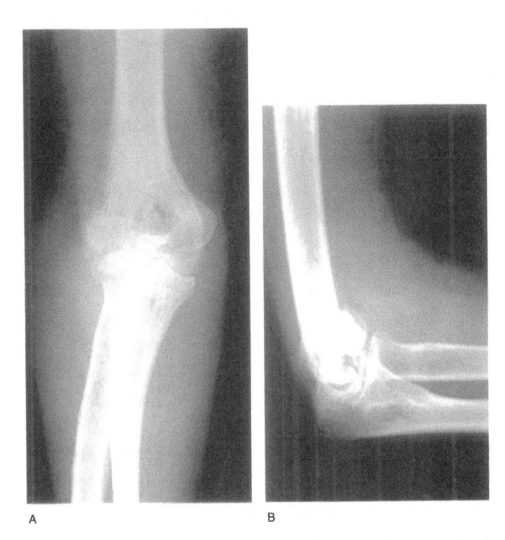

A   B

Figure 20 Case presentation of a 56-year-old woman who sustained a comminuted distal humerus fracture that was treated by total elbow arthroplasty. (A) AP and (B) lateral radiographs of a comminuted distal humeral fracture in this patient.

injury. A smaller, more recent study had 10 patients, with a mean age of 84.6, treated with a total elbow arthroplasty; using the Mayo elbow score, 8 patients had excellent results and 2 had good results with a minimum follow-up of 1 year (35).

C. Postoperative Care

Postoperative care begins with splint immobilization in a position of comfort. In most cases, the arm is splinted in 45 degrees of flexion. There are advocates of splinting in extension, since it is difficult to regain full extension after elbow surgery. However, an elbow splinted in full extension creates a very cumbersome

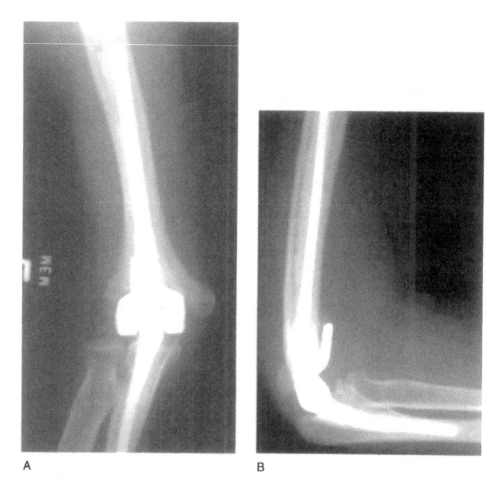

A   B

Figure 21 (A) AP and (B) lateral radiographs of patient's elbow postoperatively (same patient as in Figure 20).

position for the patient. The patient is seen 5 to 7 days postsurgery. If the wound is sealed, we begin active assisted motion. The patient is brought back a week later so that sutures and staples can be removed. Active assisted motion continues until healing is deemed imminent, based both on physical examination and a radiograph that suggests the beginning of crossing trabeculae. If the fixation looks secure and the bone is healing, passive motion is initiated. This is usually at the two- to three-month follow-up visit. Turnbuckle braces are used to help resolve persistent flexion or extension contractures.

VI. OUTCOME

Outcome in fractures of the distal humerus is usually expressed in terms of union, motion, and complications.

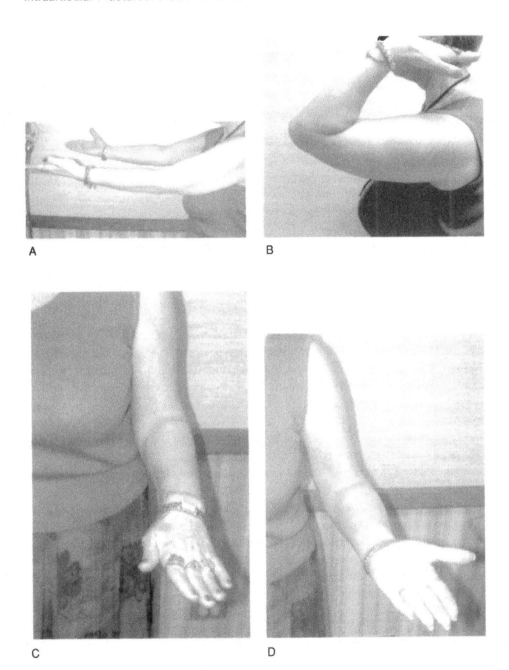

A

B

C

D

Figure 22 A-D. Patient's range of motion is demonstrated postoperatively (same patient as in Figure 20).

The rate of union for closed fractures ranges from 86 to 97% in the literature (2,11,36–38). Overall, we anticipate a healing rate for these fractures of close to 90%. The range of motion after a bicondylar fracture of the distal humerus is expected to be approximately 100 degrees in about 75% of patients (2,12,36–38). For open fractures, range of motion is generally expected to be slightly less. Complications associated with elbow fractures include stiffness, malunion, nonunion, and ulnar nerve neuropathy. Malunions and nonunions are correctable problems, as is elbow stiffness. Ulnar nerve neuropathy is frequently a difficult problem to correct. Malunions of the distal humerus can be managed with osteotomy of the distal humerus, using a posterior approach. The bone is osteotomized through the site of the previous fracture, realigned, and plated. In most cases there will be a cortical discontinuity after an osteotomy. Those discontinuities should be filled with iliac crest bone graft prior to plating. Nonunions of the distal humerus can also be managed with rigid internal fixation. In elderly patients who have suffered nonunion of a fracture, particularly a comminuted intraarticular distal humeral fracture, we recommend treatment with total elbow arthroplasty.

With regard to elbow stiffness, we have had good results in improving extension, particularly with a turnbuckle brace. In patients who do not respond well to bracing, it is possible to do elbow releases. Flexion contractures of 40 degrees or less are usually dealt with by means of an extended lateral approach. Elbows fixed in a flexed position or suffering primarily from loss of flexion are managed via an extended posterior approach. Skin flaps are raised on both the medial and lateral sides of the elbow. By splitting the extensor origin, the anterior capsule can be released. With the elbow extended, the triceps is elevated from the posterior aspect of the humerus. Medial and lateral retraction of triceps provides the exposure necessary to release the posterior capsule and clear the olecranon fossa. On the medial side, the ulnar nerve can be mobilized and the posterior medial band of the ulnar collateral ligament released to facilitate restoration of elbow flexion. Heterotopic bone can be resected at the time of release. If heterotopic bone encompasses the collateral ligaments such that they must be released, a hinged elbow fixator is placed for a period of 6 to 8 weeks. Postoperatively, patients with heterotopic bone are given indomethacin. Radiation therapy is reserved for cases of recurrent heterotopic ossification.

Management of ulnar nerve injuries can be very difficult. The ulnar nerve commonly becomes encased in scar behind the medial epicondyle after surgical treatment of a distal humeral fracture; ulnar nerve neurolysis with transposition is usually sufficient to relieve at least some of the symptoms. When the ulnar nerve is lacerated or crushed, it can be transposed and repaired. Recovery from these lesions is uniformly poor, particularly in adults.

REFERENCES

1. RS Bryan, BF Morrey. Fractures of the distal humerus. In: BF Morrey, ed. The Elbow and its Disorders, 2nd ed. Philadelphia: Saunders, 1985, pp 302–339.

2. ME Muller, S Nazarian, P Koch. AO Classification of Fractures. Berlin: Springer-Verlag, 1987.

3. JB Jupiter, DK Mehne. Fractures of the distal humerus. Orthopedics 15:825–833, 1992.

4. BJ Gainor, F Moussa, T Schott. Healing rate of transverse osteotomies used in reconstruction of distal humerus fractures. J South Orthop Assoc 4:263–268, 1995.

5. ME Baratz, JF Shanahan. Fractures of the olecranon. J South Orthop Assoc 4: 283–289, 1995.

6. CB Jones, SE Nork, J Agel, DP Hanel, MB Henley. Complications of Olecranon Osteotomies. Proceedings of the Orthopaedic Trauma Association, Vancouver, 1998.

7. KR Chin, D Ring, JB Jupiter. Double-tension-band fixation of the olecranon. Tech Shoulder Elbow Surg 1:61–66, 2000.

8. B Divelbiss, ME Baratz, W Hagberg. The triceps-sparing approach for the management of distal humerus fractures. Proceedings of the Orthopaedic Trauma Association, Vancouver, 1998.

9. ML Balk, C Manning, BH Ziran. A new triceps-splitting approach for the treatment of distal humerus fractures. Proceedings of the Orthopaedic Trauma Association, Charlotte, North Carolina, 1999.

10. H Milch. Fractures and fracture dislocations of the humeral condyles. J Trauma 4: 592–607, 1964.

11. MC Lindem. Fractures of the capitellum and trochlea. Ann Surg 76:78–82, 1922.

12. L Bohler. The Treatment of Fractures, 5th ed. New York: Grune and Stratton, 1956, pp 664–665.

13. SD Buxton. Fractures of the head of the radius and capitellum including external condylar fractures of childhood. Br Med J 2:665–666, 1936.

14. W Gejrot. On Intra-articular fractures of the capitellum and trochlea of the humerus with special reference to the treatment. Acta Chir Scand 71:253–270, 1932.

15. BT Keon-Cohen. Fractures at the elbow. J Bone Joint Surg 48A:1623–1639, 1966.

16. O Lansinger, K Mare. Fracture of the capitellum of the humerus. Ann Surg 99: 497–509, 1934.

17. RP Dushuttle, MP Coyle, JP Zawadsky, H Bloom. Fractures of the capitellum. J Trauma 25:317–321, 1985.

18. F Christopher, LF Bushnell. Conservative treatment of fracture of the capitellum. J Bone Joint Surg 17:489–492, 1935.

19. S Collert. Surgical management of fracture of the capitellum humeri. Acta Orthop Scand 48:603–606, 1977.

20. W Darrach. Open reduction of fractures of the capitellum. Ann Surg 63:487, 1916.

21. JV Fowles, MT Kassab. Fracture of the capitellum humeri. Treatment by excision. J Bone Joint Surg 56A:794–798, 1974.

22. E Alvarez, MR Patel, G Nimberg, HS Pearlman. Fracture of the capitulum humeri. J Bone Joint Surg 57A:1093–1096, 1975.

23. LA Simpson, RR Richards. Internal fixation of a capitellar fracture using Herbert screws. A case report. Clin Orthop 209:166–168, 1986.

24. RS Bryan. Fractures about the elbow in adults AAOS. Instr Course Lect 30:200–223, 1981.

25. LF Bush, EF McClain. Operative treatment of fractures of the elbow in adults AAOS. Instr Course Lect 16:265–277, 1959.

26. RR Richards, GW Khoury, FD Burke, JP Waddell. Internal fixation of capitellar

fractures using Herbert screws: A report of four cases. Can J Surg 30:188–191, 1987.

27. EL Eliason, JP North. Fractures about the elbow. Am J Surg 44:88–89, 1939.

28. WR MacAusland, ET Wyman. Fractures of the adult elbow. AAOS Instr Course Lect 24:165–181, 1975.

29. DK Mehne, J Matta. Bicolumn fractures of the adult humerus. Proceedings of American Academy of Orthopaedic Surgeons, New Orleans, 1986.

30. JB Jupiter, KA Barnes, LJ Goodman, AE Saldana. Multiplane fracture of the distal humerus. J Orthop Trauma 7:216–220, 1993.

31. EJ Riseborough, EL Radin. Intercondylar T fractures of the humerus in the adult. A comparison of operative and Non-operative treatment in twenty-nine cases. J Bone Joint Surg 51A:130–141, 1969.

32. DL Helfet, RN Hotchkiss. Internal fixation of the distal humerus: A biomechanical comparison of methods. J Orthop Trauma 4:260–264, 1990.

33. SR Jacobson, RR Glisson, JR Urbaniak. Comparison of distal humerus fracture fixation: A biomechanical study. J South Orthop Assoc 6:241–249, 1997.

34. TK Cobb, BF Morrey. Total elbow arthroplasty as primary treatment for distal humeral fractures in elderly patients. J Bone Joint Surg 79A:826–832, 1997.

35. R Gambirasio, N Riand, R Stern, P Hoffmeyer. Total elbow replacement for complex fractures of the distal humerus. An option for the elderly patient. J Bone Joint Surg 83B:974–978, 2001.

36. R Letsch, KP Schmit-Neuerburg, KM Sturmer, M Walz. Intraarticular fractures of the distal humerus: Surgical treatment and results. Clin Orthop 241:238–244, 1989.

37. DL Helfet, GJ Schmeling. Bicondylar intraarticular fractures of the distal humerus in adults. Clin Orthop 292:26–36, 1993.

38. GT Gabel, G Hanson, JB Bennett, PC Noble, HS Tullos. Intraarticular fractures of the distal humerus in the adult. Clin Orthop 216:99–108, 1987.

39. BD Browner, AM Levine, PG Trafton. Skeletal Trauma. Philadelphia: Saunders, 1998, p 1488.

5

Fractures of the Humeral Shaft

Sam Akhavan and John W. Shaffer
Case Western Reserve University/University Hospitals of Cleveland,
Cleveland, Ohio, U.S.A.

I. INTRODUCTION

Fractures of the humeral shaft account for about 3% of all fractures (1). In the majority of cases, such injuries can be treated successfully nonoperatively due to the extensive muscle and soft tissue cover that can be used to splint the fracture. In the late 1970s, Sarmiento et al. introduced a functional bracing technique that utilized soft tissue splinting while minimizing the immobilization of the elbow and shoulder, which was seen with other bracing techniques such as the hanging arm cast and thoracobrachial immobilization techniques (2–4). These techniques achieved excellent results, with rare nonunion and short healing time, in most uncomplicated humeral shaft fractures.

Despite the success of nonoperative treatments of humeral shaft fracture, indications for open reduction still abound. Option for open reduction and internal fixation include compression plating of the fracture as well as intramedullary nailing. In cases of highly comminuted fractures with segmental bone loss and open fractures with severe soft tissue injury, external fixation may also be a reasonable option. Due to the many options available in treatment, a detailed knowledge of the anatomy and function of the region is essential for proper treatment of the fracture.

II. ANATOMY AND BIOMECHANICS

The humerus is the largest bone of the upper extremity, articulating with the scapula proximally and with the radius and ulna at the elbow (Fig. 1). The shaft

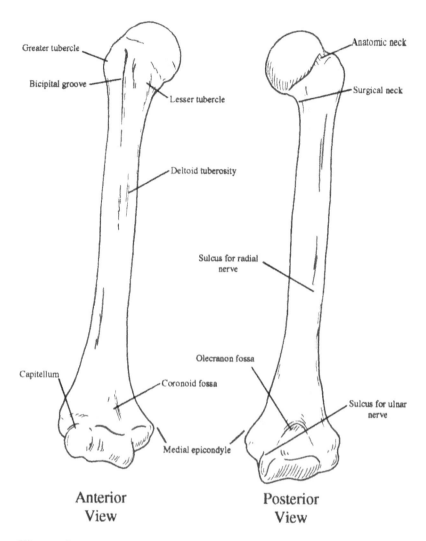

Greater tubercle
Bicipital groove
Lesser tubercle
Deltoid tuberosity
Sulcus for radial nerve
Capitellum
Coronoid fossa
Medial epicondyle
Anterior View

Anatomic neck
Surgical neck
Olecranon fossa
Sulcus for ulnar nerve
Posterior View

Figure 1 Anatomy of the human humerus. Anterior and posterior view of the humerus. (Drawn by James T. Suchy.)

of the humerus is defined as running from the upper border of the insertion of the pectoralis major to the supracondylar ridge. It is nearly cylindrical in its upper half of its extent and becomes triangular distally. It is composed of three surfaces separated by two borders (5).

The lateral border runs from the dorsal aspect of the greater tubercle to the lateral epicondyle and separates the anterolateral surface and posterior surface. It is traversed in its center by the radial nerve in its sulcus. It is the site proximally for the insertion of the teres minor and the origin of the lateral head of the triceps brachii and distally for the origin of the brachioradialis and extensor carpi radialis longus, and the insertion of the medial head of the triceps (5).

The medial border extends from the lesser tubercle to the medial epicondyle. Proximally, it is the site attachment for the teres major. Around the center is the site for the insertion of the coracobrachialis and just distal is the entrance of the nutrient canal. This canal serves as the entrance for the vascular supply of the humeral shaft, a site of crucial importance for proper healing of any fracture. In general, two-thirds of all humeri have a single nutrient. The mean position of this canal lies distal to the midpoint of the humerus and to the apex of the deltoid insertion. From this position, it spirals proximally and medially to the dorsal surface of the middle third of the shaft. This region should be avoided during any surgical operation (5,6).

Anteriorly, the surface of the humerus is divided by an oblique ridge into medial and lateral surfaces. The deltoid tuberosity, located laterally and distal to the pectoralis insertion, is an oblong area for the insertion of the deltoid. Anteromedially, it is the site for the insertion of latissimus dorsi into the intertubercular groove. Just distal and medial is the insertion of the teres minor. The middle of the shaft contains a rough surface for the coracobrachialis and the distal part is flat and smooth, giving origin to the brachialis (5).

The musculature of the humeral shaft provides a natural splinting mechanism and may be a major factor contributing to the success of closed methods for the treatment of most fractures. When an operation is required, all approaches to the humeral shaft have the potential for dangerous outcome due to the extensive neurovascular structures.

A. Nerves

Injuries to the radial nerve are among the most common complications of injuries to the humeral shaft. The nerve is a continuation of the posterior cord of the brachial plexus and incorporates fibers of the C5 to T1 nerve roots (Fig. 2). It supplies the extensor muscles of the arm and forearm as well as the sensation to the overlying skin. It courses deep to the axillary artery at the shoulder, crossing the tendon of the latissimus dorsi, and then passes between the long head of the triceps muscle and the shaft of the humerus beneath the teres major. The nerve then courses in the spiral groove on the posterior aspect of the humerus in between the two heads of triceps before crossing the back of the humerus and piercing the lateral intermuscular septum. It then crosses the elbow in the anterior compartment, lying in between the brachioradialis and brachialis muscle. It is responsible for innervating the triceps, brachioradialis, extensor carpi radialis longus, extensor carpi radialis brevis, and the anconeus in the arm (5,7).

The radial nerve is most vulnerable with fractures of the midshaft of the humerus, as it lies on the back of the bone in the spiral groove. During surgery, this position makes the nerve vulnerable to damage by drills, taps, and screws inserted when an anterior plate is applied to the middle third of the bone. In addition, dissection of the distal third of the humerus may also damage the nerve as it lies in between the brachioradialis and brachialis. Splitting the brachialis along its midline during this dissection may provide a cushion and act to protect the nerve (7).

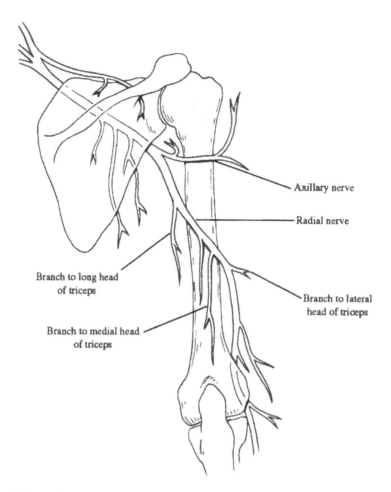

Figure 2 Course of the radial nerve. Posterior view of the humerus outlining the course of the radial nerve as it branches from the posterior cord. The course is highlighted posteriorly as it crosses the midshaft of the humerus, where it is most vulnerable in fractures. (Drawn by James T. Suchy.)

The median nerve originates from the medial and lateral cord of the brachial plexus and incorporates fibers of the C6 to T1 nerve roots. It courses through the arm along with the brachial artery, anteromedial to the humerus. It originally starts lateral to the artery but crosses the artery in the middle/distal part of the arm and finishes medial at the elbow, where it can be found superficial to the brachialis muscle (5,7).

The ulnar nerve is a terminal branch of the medial cord and includes fibers from the C8 and T1 spinal roots. It is initially medial and posterior to the axillary and eventually the brachial artery. At the level of the midshaft, it angles dorsally to enter the posterior compartment via the medial intermuscular septum. It then follows the medial head of the triceps muscle to the groove behind the medial epicondyle. In this position, it lies only below skin and fascia and can be readily palpated. It is most vulnerable during dissections of the lower third of the arm, where it lies deep to the medial head of triceps. To prevent damage to the nerve, it is recommended that any elevation of the triceps be done only in the subperiosteal plane (5,7).

B. Arteries

The three arteries of the humeral shaft all branch off the brachial artery and anastamose freely around the elbow joint (Fig. 3). In the arm, each artery runs along with its associated nerve.

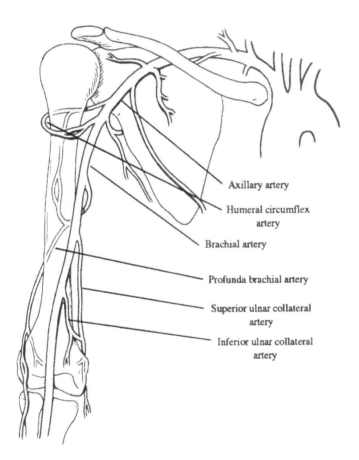

Axillary artery

Humeral circumflex
artery

Brachial artery

Profunda brachial artery

Superior ulnar collateral
artery

Inferior ulnar collateral
artery

Figure 3 Arterial supply of the humerus. Anterior view of the humerus and its blood supply. Special attention can be paid to the profunda brachii as it courses posteriorly alongside the radial nerve. The brachial artery runs together with the medial nerve while the superior ulnar collateral artery runs with the ulnar nerve. (Drawn by James T. Suchy.)

The brachial artery is a continuation of the axillary artery and begins at the lower border of the teres major. It follows a medial course along with the medial nerve, where it can be readily palpated. Distally, it curves to the front of the arm and lies in between the two epicondyles at the antecubital fossa.

The deep brachial artery branches off the brachial artery proximally, just distal to the lower border of the teres major muscle. The artery courses posteriorly with the radial nerve, in between the long and lateral head of the triceps.

Finally, the superior ulnar collateral branches off just distal to the midshaft of the humerus. It runs through the medial intermuscular septum and descends with the ulnar nerve on the surface of the medial head of triceps.

C. Biomechanics

The biomechanics of the humeral shaft are similar to those of most long bones and are affected strongly by the surrounding muscles. In addition, the non-weight-bearing nature of the humerus makes force distribution seen by the bone unique and may be partially responsible for the common fracture patterns.

The shaft of the humerus is stronger in compression than either end of the bone. It is therefore fairly uncommon to see shaft fractures due to purely compressive forces, as are seen in falls on the outstretched hand or directly on the arm. These types of mechanisms are more likely to lead to a proximal humeral fracture. In contrast, the proximal and distal aspects of the humerus are much less likely to react to bending or torsional forces due to the presence of multiaxial joint at the shoulder and elbow. These types of forces are much more likely to be transmitted through the shaft of the humerus (3,8).

Klenerman in 1969 studied the biomechanical effect of different forces on the fracture patterns seen in the humerus. Bending forces, applied to the midshaft, tended to result in a transverse pattern with about a 20% incidence of cracks preparatory to the separation of a butterfly fragment. Klenerman surmised that muscle forces in vivo might well have led to the separation of the butterfly fragment. Torsional forces, on the other hand, led to a spiral fracture pattern. In comparing experimental and clinical fractures, he found a higher incidence of middle- and distal-third fractures clinically than seen experimentally. This may well be due to the presence of the deltoid and pectoralis proximally and their role in stabilizing the proximal humerus in torsion, thus conferring the forces more distally (8).

The location of the shaft fracture may affect the pull of the fragments by the surrounding musculature (Fig. 4A to D). A fracture located above the pectoral insertion will have the proximal fragment pulled into abduction by the rotator cuff musculature, mainly the supraspinatus. A fracture below the pectoralis insertion would lead to the proximal fragment being pulled into adduction by the pectoralis, while the distal fragment would be pulled into abduction by the deltoid. A fracture below both the deltoid and the pectoralis would lead to the proximal fragment being pulled into abduction, mainly by the deltoid (8,9).

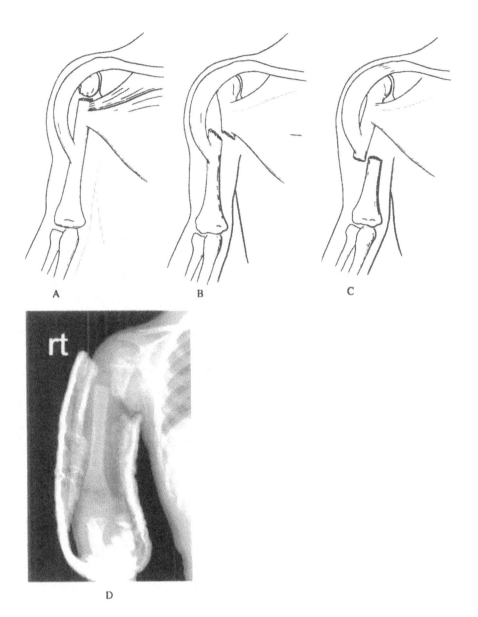

Figure 4   Fracture patterns of the humeral shaft. The pattern of the fracture can be predicted based on the location of the fracture and the pull of the deltoid, pectoralis major and rotator cuff muscles. A. Proximal fractures will have the proximal fragment pulled into abduction due to the pull of the rotator cuff muscles. B. Fractures below the pectoralis major insertion will have the proximal fragment pulled into adduction by the pectoralis, while the distal fragment is pulled into abduction by the deltoid. C. Fractures below the deltoid insertion will have a proximal fragment pulled into abduction by the deltoid. D. X-ray of a 2-year-old girl following a fall with a humeral shaft fracture pattern similar to that seen in Fig. 4B due to the location of the fracture. (Drawn by James T. Suchy.)

III. CLASSIFICATION

There are no universally accepted classification systems for humeral shaft fractures. Müller's alphanumeric system for classification of long bone fractures may be used. This classification scheme uses the letters A, B, and C to group fractures as simple, wedge, and complex fractures, respectively. Each group is then further divided into three subgroups based on the severity of the fracture. This method was intended to simplify the classification and allow for uniform system of classification. No treatment protocols have been formulated for this classification system, although the more severe fractures tend to have poorer prognosis (10).

In general, an accurate description of the fracture should involve its anatomical location, the type of fracture, and any associated soft tissue injuries. The mechanism of injury may be helpful in distinguishing between high- and low-energy fractures. The location of the fracture may be divided into three categories: above the pectoralis insertion, below the pectoralis but above the deltoid insertion, or below both muscle insertions. This distinction may be helpful in determining the deforming biomechanics of these muscles, as described above.

Open fractures of the humeral shaft are classified under the Gustillo system, where a grade I indicates a wound of less than 1 cm and a relatively low-energy injury, a grade II indicates a wound greater than 1 cm with a moderate-energy injury and soft tissue damage, and a grade III indicates a high-energy fracture with extensive soft tissue damage or a traumatic amputation (11). The presence of a neurovascular injury may be a further indication for surgery, as it may dictate a need for stable reduction of the fracture to protect the repair of the nerve or artery.

IV. DIAGNOSIS (TABLE 1)

In evaluating patients with suspected humeral shaft fractures, special attention should be paid to the mechanism of injury. In the majority of cases, a high-

Table 1   Diagnosis and Workup of Humeral Shaft Fracture

History and physical examination
    Mechanism of injury: high-energy vs. low-energy
    Pain, swelling, and deformity
    Crepitation at fracture site
    Neuromuscular examination: motor/sensory
    Vascular examination
    Check for compartment syndrome
    Check for associated injuries
    Past medical history, medications/allergies
Radiological evaluation
    Anteroposterior and lateral view of humerus
    Views of elbow and shoulder including axillary if dislocation suspected

versus a low-energy mechanism may be determined by history alone. Low-energy fractures, such as falls on the arm and twisting injuries, are less likely to have associated injuries. In the evaluation of high-energy injuries, as can be seen from motor vehicle accidents, a thorough examination of the entire body is crucial.

Most patients upon presentation will have the traditional symptoms of a fracture, such as pain, swelling, deformity, and crepitations. The arm may also be shortened and hypermobile at the site of the fracture. A thorough evaluation of the neurovascular status of the injured extremity is crucial. Motor strength should be tested both proximally and distally to ensure that no injury to the radial, median, or ulnar nerve is missed. The compartments of the arm should also be evaluated to make sure that no compartment syndrome is present. All abrasions and wounds should be probed for the possibility of an open injury, which may warrant the need for emergent surgery.

If surgery is a consideration in the treatment of the patient, an evaluation of the patient's medical status should be performed in the initial setting, including all laboratory and imaging studies.

Radiological examination of the fracture should include anteroposterior (AP) and lateral views of the humerus. These views should be obtained at 90 degrees to each other to ensure proper characterization of any fracture displacement. If the lesion is not accurately assessed by the humerus film, separate views of the elbow and shoulder should also be obtained. If a dislocation is suspected at the shoulder, an axillary view should also be included. In pathological fractures, more thorough evaluation with staging examinations may be necessary to determine the extent of disease.

V. NONOPERATIVE MANAGEMENT

The biomechanics of the humerus and its surrounding tissues make it readily reducible. The free movement of the scapulohumeral joint minimizes torsional stresses through the bone, making rigid immobilization unnecessary for proper healing (3). In addition, the humerus acts mostly as a lever, with little or no weight-bearing function or compressive forces. The influence of gravity places the fracture fragments in a physiologically dependent position, which facilitates reduction (3).

Many techniques have been attempted in the past. Initially, thoracoacromial immobilization with the use of a cast or a sling and swath was used to splint the fractured extremity against the thorax. The rationale for these techniques was to provide stability to the fracture site. The cast or swath was applied for 3 to 4 weeks, after which the patient was switched to a lighter sling. Beside the obvious problem of prolonged immobilization of the shoulder and elbow, this technique did not make use of gravity to help place the fracture in a dependent position. As a result, it was rarely been used since the advent of function bracing (3).

Caldwell in 1933 introduced the hanging cast as a method of providing stability to the fracture while also placing traction on the fracture fragments by the use of gravity. The technique involved placing a cast from the axilla to the hand, with the elbow held at 90 degrees of flexion and the forearm in midpronation. The upper portion of the cast was adjusted to account for the location of the fracture and its surrounding biomechanics. Further investigation led to slight modification in the cast, including changing the length of the sling aids to adjust for posterior versus anterior bowing and changing the position of the suspension hook so as to correct for medial versus lateral bowing as well as to change the amount of traction on the fracture fragments. Although good results were achieved with this method, the cast was generally uncomfortable and had to be maintained in a dependent position. In addition, an improperly applied or heavy cast could lead to distraction of the fracture site (2).

The short brachial splint, also known as a coaptation or U splint, is a modification on the hanging cast method while still using gravity to provide traction on the fracture fragments. A molded plaster slab is placed around the elbow and extended over the elbow. It is then held in place by an elastic bandage with the forearm suspended by use of a felt wrist cuff. This splinting method is still used today in emergency rooms as a method of temporary splinting. When used as the definitive form of treatment, however, results have not been superior to functional bracing (3,12).

The functional brace (Fig. 5A to C) introduced by Sarmiento in the late 1970s has become the treatment of choice for closed treatment of humeral shaft fractures. This method uses both gravity to align the fractured segments as well as physiologically induced motion to promote osteogenesis. The brace acts to stiffen the soft tissue, providing a splinting effect to the fracture fragment. It does not, however, immobilize the fracture site. As a result, fractures of the humerus treated with functional bracing tend to have some degree of varus angulation, but they are still acceptable both cosmetically and functionally (4).

Unlike the hanging cast or the U splint, the functional brace does not immobilize either the shoulder or the elbow joint. The adjustable brace is tightened around the soft tissues surrounding the fracture site and the arm is allowed to hang freely to the side in a normal position. The brace does not actually have to cover every one of the fracture fragments as long as the soft tissues are compressed. This creates an ideal environment for fracture healing.

The functional brace may be used for almost all closed fractures, with union rates of greater than 90% (4,13–15). The fracture geometry and location have little effect on healing as long as the soft tissue envelope is intact. Even open fractures with little surrounding soft tissue injury (Gustillo II and lower) may be treated successfully as long as thorough irrigation and antibiotic treatment are undertaken. Obesity in and of itself is not a contraindication to functional bracing, although these fractures do tend to have a higher level of angular deformity (14).

Some humeral shaft fractures may not be good candidates for functional bracing. These include closed or open fractures with significant soft tissue dam-

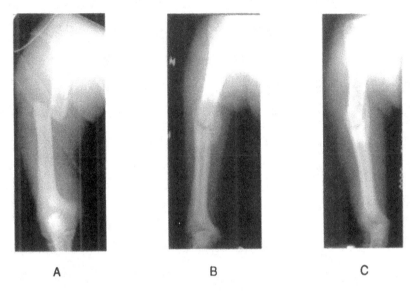

A   B   C

Figure 5 Fracture bracing of humeral shaft fractures. 17-year-old male s/p football injury with a humeral shaft fracture treated with fracture bracing. A. AP x-ray taken in emergency room. B. AP x-ray after treatment with a functional brace for 8 weeks. C. AP x-ray of the same fracture after functional bracing for 3 months. (X-rays provided by Heather A. Vallier, MD, Metrohealth Medical Center, Cleveland, Ohio, U.S.A.)

age. As the soft tissue envelope is crucial for splinting of the fracture fragments, these fractures will tend to have a higher rate of nonunion or unacceptable angular deformity. In addition, patients with polytrauma or bilateral fractures will also tend to have a higher level of angular deformity. Fractures associated with vascular injury that requires repair of the vessel will need to undergo open reduction and internal fixation of the fracture to protect the repair.

Application of the functional brace must be delayed, as the patient may initially have too much and pain and swelling for proper application. These patients may first be treated with either a hanging cast or a coaptation splint. As soon as symptoms allow, the functional brace is fitted and placed. The cylindrical sleeve should begin about 2 cm distal to the axilla and terminate about 2 cm proximal to the humeral condyles. The treatment regiment is started as soon as symptoms allow. The patient is encouraged initially to partake in range-of-motion exercises, especially at the elbow, with particular emphasis on extension. Shoulder exercises should be limited to pendulums only, as active abduction and elevation of the arm may lead to the development of angular deformities. The brace in most studies is usually be removed by about 10 to 13 weeks, or when union of the fracture is confirmed both radiographically and clinically (4,14). Most studies show excellent results with these methods, with nonunion rates comparable to those from open fixation, at about 1 to 6% (4,13–16).

VI. OPERATIVE TREATMENT

While most humeral shaft fractures can be successfully treated by nonoperative methods, several types of fractures warrant open reduction and internal fixation. When such indications do arise, several treatment options are available. The main decision in considering open reduction involves plating of the fracture versus intramedullary nailing. Much controversy still exist as to whether one method is truly superior; in most cases, the decision comes down to the surgeon's personal preference and his or her level of comfort with a particular procedure.

A. Indications (9,12,14,15,17,18) (Table 2)

In considering which fracture pattern may require open reduction, several principles must be considered. The key to the success of closed treatment of humeral shaft fractures is an intact soft tissue envelope to act as a splint for the fracture fragments. If this envelope is violated or disrupted, the use of functional bracing will very likely lead to nonunion or an unacceptable deformity. Therefore it is widely accepted that type III open injuries and even type II injuries with significant soft tissue damage (as may occur from a gunshot wound) are more likely to be successfully treated by plating or nailing of the fracture.

In addition, polytrauma patients who are bed-bound and unable to sit up are not good candidates for functional bracing as they are unable to benefit from the effect of gravity to reduce the fracture fragments. Patients with associated ipsilateral forearm fractures (the "floating elbow") will also not truly benefit from functional bracing due to the inherent instability of this fracture pattern and should have both fractures fixed at the same time. Patients with bilateral fractures should also be treated operatively so as to promote earlier recovery and mobilization.

Failure of closed treatments should also warrant open fixation. Many authors have studied the outcome of closed treatments, with special consideration to varus angulation. There have been no adverse functional effects seen with varus deformities in excess of 30 degrees. However, any angulation of greater than 15 degrees will usually result in an expressible deformity. Klenerman showed

Table 2   Indications for Surgical Treatment

Open fractures with significant soft tissue injuries (type II and greater)
Bed-bound polytrauma patients
Ipsilateral forearm fracture ("floating elbow")
Bilateral fractures
Failed closed treatment
Neurovascular injury requiring complications
Pathological fractures
Relative indication
Obese patient

that the humerus can accommodate up to 20 degrees of anterior angulation, 30 degrees of varus angulation, and 3 cm of shortening without any loss of function, strength, or cosmesis (19). Obese patients, although more difficult to treat by closed methods, are also better able to conceal greater degrees of deformity.

Other indications for operative treatment include associated nerve and vascular injury. With the repair of the neurovascular structures, it is recommended that a formal approach and repair of the fracture be undertaken so as to protect the repair. Finally, pathological fractures, especially those involving poor bone stock or impending potential fractures, should also be treated operatively.

External fixation may also be used as a method of operative fixation of humeral shaft fractures. Indications for external fixation are limited to highly comminuted fractures or fractures with significant soft tissue damage. Management with external fixation may also allow for quick stabilization of the fracture in patients unable to tolerate a formal internal fixation.

B. Compression Plating

Compression plating (Fig. 6A to E) is the preferred method of fixation at our institution for most humeral shaft fractures (Table 3). Most surgeons prefer the use of an anterolateral approach to expose the humeral shaft. One of the major advantages of such an exposure is that it allows for identification and protection of the radial nerve. This approach involves an incision over the lateral border of the biceps about 10 cm proximal to the flexion crease of the elbow. After medial retraction of the biceps, the radial nerve must be identified in between the brachi-

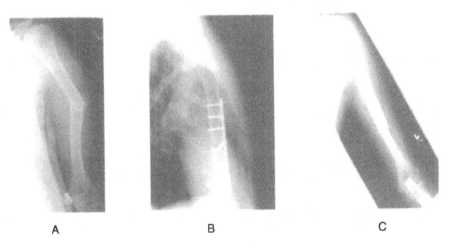

A   B   C

Figure 6   Plating of humeral shaft fractures. 38-year-old male following a motor vehicle accident with a humeral shaft fracture treated operatively with plating. A. Preoperative AP X-ray demonstrating a below-the-deltoid-insertion fracture pattern. B. Postoperative film of the same fracture treated by plating with lag screw placement. C. AP view of same fracture at 3 months.

Table 3 Advantages to Plating

Exploration and protection of radial nerve
Visualization of fracture site
Established good results
Less shoulder and elbow problems than with intramedullary nailing

alis and brachioradialis muscles just above the elbow and followed proximally until in pierces the intermuscular septum. While carefully staying medial to the radial nerve, the brachialis can then be incised longitudinally and the humerus exposed (1,7,9,12,14,18).

Alternatively, a posterior approach through the triceps muscle can also be used for exposure of distal humeral shaft fractures. This exposure does not involve any true internervous plane, as both heads of triceps are innervated by the radial nerve. The nerve inserts relatively close to the origin of the heads and then lies within the substance of the muscle. A longitudinal split of triceps therefore does not affect the innervation, especially in the medial head, which is dually innervated by the radial and ulnar nerves. Initial dissection involves splitting the lateral and long head of triceps bluntly proximally and sharply distally. Below this plane will lie the medial or deep head of triceps, which, once split, will reveal the humeral shaft. During this dissection, two main dangers exist. First, the radial nerve lies in the spiral groove, which is above the origin of the medial triceps. Identification of the nerve during dissection will prevent any inadvertent injury. Second, The ulnar nerve lies below the medial head of triceps. It is therefore crucial that any elevation of the triceps muscle be done in a subperiosteal plane in order to avoid damage (1,9,12,14,18).

Following exposure of the fracture site, the hematoma is evacuated and the fracture fragments are debrided. The choice of instrumentation has been a point of controversy over the years. Originally, most authors advocated the use of a broad 4.5-mm dynamic compression plate (DCP), so as to allow for angulation of the cortex screws. The goal of this angulation was to prevent any further splitting of the humerus, which was seen when all the screws were placed in line. The use of a broad plate, however, has several disadvantages, including excessive soft tissue stripping and poor fit of the plate on the shaft, especially in patients with small arms. Some authors have recently advocated the use of a narrow 4.5-mm DCP plate and even a 3.5-mm plate with similar results as those seen with the broader plate (12,17,20).

Following placement of the plate, most authors advocate the placement of at least six cortical screws above and below the fracture site, with many recommending eight in more complicated fractures. The plate may be bent to better conform to the contours of the humerus and provide better plate-bone contact. The screws should be angled to prevent the above-mentioned splitting, which can be seen when all screws are in line. If severe comminution with bone loss is seen, bone grafting can be used to fill in any defects (20,25).

Results from plating of fractures have generally been excellent, with most authors quoting union rates of 94 to 100% (13,17,20–25). In general, when non-union does occur, it tends to occur with fractures at the junction of the middle and distal thirds of the humeral shaft. This may well be due to the vascular supply of the humerus and the location of the main nutrient foramina (5,6,26).

The main determinant of success lies in shoulder motion. Functional range of motion has usually restored in more than 80% of patients. In most cases where shoulder motion is limited following plate fixation, associated severe soft tissue and skeletal injuries are usually present (9,22,23,27).

The major complication of plate fixation involves radial nerve injury. The radial nerve is vulnerable both during initial exposure and during placement of the cortical screws. In addition, several authors have reported neuropraxias attributed to excessive traction during fixation of the fracture. In all cases, these injuries were temporary and healed fully (17,20,22,27–30).

C. Intramedullary Nailing

Over the course of the past several years, intramedullary nailing (Fig. 7A to F) has gained great favor among many orthopedic surgeons for the fixation of many different types of fractures (Table 4). While the initial results achieved in humeral shaft fractures were not as favorable as those seen with plating, recent technological improvements in the nail have led to renewed interest in intramedullary nailing. Due to the many different types of nails available as well as techniques for insertion, the decision process making for nailing of humeral shaft fractures must involve detailed knowledge of the fracture type, location, and properties as well as an awareness of the native properties of the bone, including canal size and shape.

There are many theoretical advantages to using intramedullary nails in the fixation of humeral shaft fractures. First, the relatively noninvasive nature of the surgery preserves the fracture site. The fracture hematoma is not violated, which may enhance healing and reduce the incidence of infection. In addition, the surgery can usually be performed through a small incision with little blood loss. The surgery does not involve a lot of soft tissue stripping, which may preserve the vascularity of the bone and also enhance healing. Finally, patients who will require the arm for weight bearing postoperatively (such as polytrauma patients) are able to put weight on the affected extremity immediately after surgery (18,22, 27,31–33).

There are several contraindications to nailing of humeral shaft fractures. First, very distal or proximal fractures that leave small, short fragments of bone will not allow for good fixation of the fracture site. Second, where there is pre-existing deformity of the canal, passage of the nail may not be possible. Finally, children with open physes and adolescents are also not good candidate (32,34).

The choice of insertion method has come under much debate in the past few years. Retrograde insertion is ideal for fractures of the proximal and middle thirds, while antegrade insertion applies more to fractures of the middle and

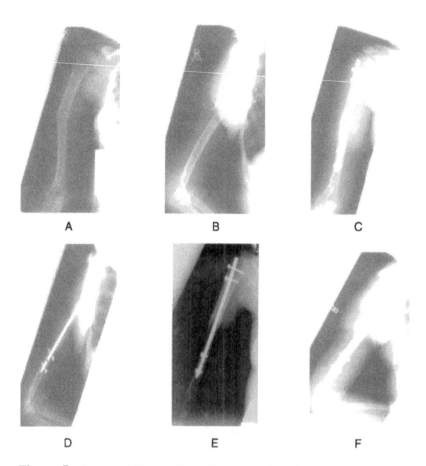

A   B   C

D   E   F

Figure 7   Intramedullary nailing of humeral shaft fractures. Fiftyfive-year-old female with history of breast cancer found to have metastatic disease to the right humerus. A and B. Preoperative AP and lateral x-rays demonstrating a pathological fracture of the humeral shaft. C and D. AP and lateral x-rays of the same fracture after intramedullary nailing at 10 months. E and F. AP and lateral x-rays of the same fracture at 1 year. (X-rays provided by Patrick J. Getty, M.D., University Hospitals of Cleveland.)

distal third. Much controversy still exists when a choice needs to be made between the two. Many authors originally inserted intramedullary devices antegrade, either through or lateral to the rotator cuff insertion. Although good unions were achieved with this method and few intraoperative complications were seen, many patients' postoperative course was complicated by limitations of shoulder function. In addition, some authors have reported complications secondary to the nail backing out proximally, requiring a second operation for removal of hardware (22,27,33,35,36).

As a result, many recent reports are advocating the use of a retrograde portal for nail insertion. Two such portals can be used. The first is an olecranon portal, which is created in the proximal slope of the olecranon fossa. The second

Table 4   Advantages of Intramedullary Nailing

Preservation of the fracture site
Intact fracture hematoma
Reduced risk of infection
Small incision with reduced blood loss
Preserve vascularity of fracture site
Immediate postoperative weight bearing
Contraindications
Very proximal/distal fractures
Predeformed or small canal
Children with open physes

is a metaphyseal portal, created in the center of the distal metaphyseal triangle, about 2 cm proximal to the olecranon fossa. Although both techniques have achieved similar results in terms of union and shoulder and elbow function, proponents of the olecranon technique state that this approach is more line with the axis of the humeral shaft and therefore requires less reaming of the anterior cortex. The metaphyseal technique, in contrast, requires more reaming for insertion of the nail but does not violate the elbow capsule, which may reduce the incidence of elbow dysfunction (18,33,35).

While reasonable success has been achieved with both types of portals, both do weaken the biomechanical property of the native bone. Strohman et al. demonstrated that the creation of a distal portal in the human humerus, whether through the olecranon or the metaphysis, reduced the resistance to torque by more than 50% and the load to failure by about 20% when compared to intact bone. While intact bones subjected to these stresses fractured proximally to the olecranon, those specimens with portals fractured either through the anterior cortex opposite the portal or through the portal itself. These results are indicative of an iatrogenic weakness that is created in the bone, a factor that may be important if the arm is to be used for weight bearing postoperatively (33).

Several different types of nails are available. The use of flexible nails (Fig. 8A and B) has largely fallen out of favor because of to the multitude of locked nails available and the success of such devices in other long bones of the body. Of the devices currently available, the Ender nail is the most popular and most often used. This device is made of stainless steel and is available in a 3.5-mm diameter for the humerus. It is composed of a beveled tip and a flattened eyelet at the head for insertion and extraction. It can be inserted both antegrade or retrograde, depending on the fracture type, the surgeon's preference, and the fracture pattern. Results from flexible nails demonstrate union rates of 92 to 99% depending on the type of nail and the technique (31,37–39).

Flexible nails confer stability to the fracture axially but are deficient in rotational stability. In addition, the nails may back out from the portal of insertion, requiring a second operation for removal. To a degree, this complication

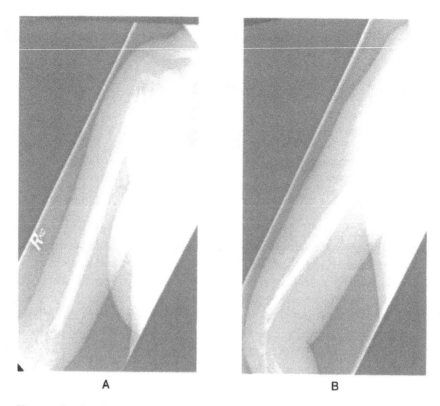

A   B

Figure 8   Intramedullary nailing of humeral shaft fractures. Sixteen-year-old female 5 years following a humeral shaft fracture treated with flexible intramedullary nails. A and B. AP and lateral views of the now healed fracture.

may be avoided by fixating the insertion site with the use of a wire. With Ender nails, this may be achieved by inserting the wire through the proximal eyelet.

Because of these shortcomings, most authors are now advocating the use of locked rigid nails. Many different types of the nails are available with a variety of proximal and distal fixation options and angles. These nails may also be inserted either antegrade or retrograde. One of the major improvements in the past years has been the development of nails of various sizes for intramedullary nailing. The original rigid nail devices were all of uniform size, requiring reaming for proper insertion; but more recent nails have smaller diameters and do not require reaming. The original Seidel nail has a distal fin that would anchor into the bone on expansion. It also has slots both proximally and distally for placement of locking screws. Several problems with this device have been reported. Robinson et al. reported a 30% incidence of improper expansion of the distal fins in 30 humeral fractures. In addition, he also reported failure to properly place one or both proximal locking screws in 8 of 30 fractures due to complications with the guidance device (40).

While initial results of intramedullary nailing were somewhat discouraging, especially in light of the high success rate of plating, the more recently developed rigid nails have shown results fairly comparable to those of plating. The Russell-Taylor nail as well as several other custom rigid nails have yielded excellent results. Chapman et al., in a comparison between plating and use of Russell-Taylor nails, showed union rates of 93 and 87%, respectively, at 16 weeks, a difference that was not significant (22). Other authors have reported similar union rates, ranging from 88 to 95% (36,38,41).

Significant infections are rare with humeral shaft fractures owing to the excellent vascular supply and the soft tissue envelope of the fracture. As mentioned earlier, one of the theoretical advantages of intramedullary nailing in closed fractures would be a lower rate of infection, because the fracture site is left undisturbed. In general, most studies show similar infection rates, ranging from 0 to 6.7%—numbers that are comparable to those reported from plating (21–23,30,34,36,37,40–42).

Due to the similar rates of union and infections, most authors gauge the success of surgery in humeral shaft fractures on the basis of shoulder function. The intramedullary nail was originally inserted through the rotator cuff, with the cuff then repaired over the insertion site. Stern et al., in 60 humeral shaft fractures stabilized by rush rods, had a 56% incidence of adhesive capsulitis (41). In this series, most nails were inserted through the rotator cuff. Brumback et al. advocated inserting the nail lateral and distal to the supraspinatus insertion to avoid shoulder dysfunction (37). While no studies have specifically looked at not violating the rotator cuff and the resulting shoulder dysfunction, most authors will agree that proper identification of the supraspinatus tendon and its eventual splitting in the well-vascularized zone, rather than the relatively avascular zone in the 1-cm zone prior to its insertion at the greater trochanter, will lead to better healing and subsequently superior shoulder function (43). Finally, during insertion of an antegrade nail, special attention should be paid to burying the nail so as to prevent impingement.

The use of retrograde nailing may provide better functional outcomes in shoulder function. The use of the olecranon portal, as previously described, violates the elbow capsule and in theory may affect elbow function (33,35). Lin, in a series of 48 humeral shaft fractures, performed the nailing in a retrograde manner using both the metaphyseal and the olecranon portals. He achieved excellent elbow motion in 47 of 48 patients, with no statistical difference between the two methods (35). In general, good recovery of both shoulder and elbow function may be related more to a good postoperative program with special attention paid to regaining movement at both the elbow and shoulder than to the entry portal that has been used.

D.   External Fixation

While the indications for external fixation are limited, given the success of other methods of stabilization, several situations do warrant its use. First, there are cases where severe soft tissue injuries are present, which limit the surgeon's ability to safely fix the fracture by internal means, and, second, there are cases where segmental bone loss is present. Additionally, in the presence of a vascular injury, external fixation may provide a quick and stable fixation method to allow for emergent repair of the injury. Recently, some authors have also advocated the use of external fixation in highly comminuted high-velocity gunshot wound injuries, with excellent results (44,45).

In all cases, the use of an external fixator does not provide definitive treatment of the fracture. After initial stabilization and soft tissue management, the external fixator is removed in exchange for either functional bracing or internal fixation.

VII. SURGICAL TECHNIQUES

A. Plating Techniques

The choice of incision and approach to the humeral shaft is dependent on the location of the fracture and any associated injury, such as the need to explore for a radial nerve injury. Traditionally, most surgeons will perform an anterolateral approach for a fracture of the proximal two-thirds and a posterior approach for a distal third fracture.

In an anterolateral approach, the patient is placed supine on the table with a towel or pad under the shoulder to support the scapula. The arm in then abducted and draped free from the sterile sheets. The coracoid process, deltopectoral interval, lateral bicipital sulcus, and lateral epicondyle are identified and may be marked out. Following incision, the deltopectoral interval is explored with protection of the cephalic vein to expose the humerus proximally. As the dissection proceeds distally, the brachialis muscle is identified and split medially, thus preserving its innervation laterally by the radial nerve and medially by the musculocutaneous nerve. In addition, lateral retraction of the brachialis will protect the radial nerve. To further facilitate the placement of a plate, the arm is flexed at the elbow and the anterior portion of the deltoid attachment as well as the origin of the brachialis may be detached. Besides the radial nerve, the lateral antebrachial cutaneous nerve must be protected medially during this approach.

In a posterior approach, the patient is placed prone on the table and the arm is abducted 90 degrees over an elbow rest. The arm is then draped free. The surface landmarks—the posterior edge of the acromion and the olecranon process—are then identified and marked out. Following incision, the posterior border of the deltoid is identified and the fascia divided. The dissection then proceeds between the long and lateral head of the triceps. This approach will expose the radial nerve as well as the profunda brachii artery and its branches; great care must be taken not to injure them as the dissection proceeds, or from retraction. The medial head of the triceps can then be split distally to fully expose the shaft of the humerus. Other structures to consider during this dissection are the lateral brachial cutaneous nerve during the initial exposure and the axillary nerve and posterior humeral circumflex proximally.

Following exposure of the humeral shaft and evacuation of the hematoma, the fragments are reduced anatomically and lag-screw fixation is attempted. A 4.5-mm plate is then used and bent to approximate the contour of the humeral shaft. The choice of a broad versus a narrow plate is dependent on the shape and size of the bone, although good results have been achieved with both. In a transverse fracture, the plate should be placed in compression if possible. With other fracture types, the plate is applied in neutralization to protect the lag-screw construct.

B. Intramedullary (IM) Nailing Technique

Two different techniques are currently available for intramedullary nailing of humeral shaft fractures. The choice of which to use is dependent on the comfort level of the surgeon as well as the location of the fracture. In general, the ante-grade nailing method is used mostly for fractures of the middle and distal thirds of the humeral shaft, while the retrograde approach may be used for more proximal fractures. In either case, careful preoperative imaging and positioning of the fluoroscopic C arm is crucial to obtain proper imaging of the fracture fragments and their orientation as well as to make sure that the fracture is reducible.

The antegrade approach involves accessing the intramedullary canal through the shoulder, along the lateral junction of the articular cartilage and the lateral third of the humeral head, approximately 1 cm medial to the greater tuberosity. To achieve this access, a 4-cm incision is made anterolateral to the acromion, overlying the deltoid. The deltoid is then split and the subdeltoid bursa identified and removed to expose the supraspinatus tendon. Some authors have recommended a formal exposure to the rotator cuff so as to make sure that its fibers are split along the more vascular portion (just lateral to the articular surface) rather than in the proximal portion 1 cm from its insertion on the greater tuberosity, where the vascularity is poor. The tendon is then split along it fibers and the previously mentioned insertion site exposed.

Following this exposure, a guidewire may be inserted through the entry portal under direct visualization. The size of the nail and proper position of the canal are determined in this manner. The canal can then be reamed to the proper-size nail. The nail is then inserted with great care being taken not to violate the cortex of the canal. The surgeon must be sure that the nail is properly buried in the humeral head so that no impingement results from a proud nail.

The proximal locking screws may then be inserted, with the aid of the guidewire, from lateral to medial. In doing so, excessive violation of the medial cortex may place the axillary nerve at risk due to rotation of the proximal fragment. The distal screws may be placed in a freehand manner either anterior to posterior or lateral to medial. In the prior case, the lateral antebrachial cutaneous nerve may be at risk, whereas the radial nerve may come into play with lateral-to-medial screw placement, especially if the tip of the nail lies proximal to the end of the canal.

The retrograde approach has been advocated as a potential alternative to violating the rotator cuff, with less resulting limitation of shoulder function. The two commonly used portals of entry and their advantages were discussed previously. This technique is usually not advocated for distal third fractures.

The patient is most commonly placed supine, although prone and lateral approaches have also been described. The arm is crossed over the chest and placed on an arm board. A longitudinal incision is made over the triceps insertion distally, and the triceps is split proximal to the olecranon but well distal to the radial groove. The ulnar nerve is located medially and the radial nerve laterally during this approach, although these nerves are rarely encountered. As previously mentioned, the olecranon portal is more in line with the canal of the humeral shaft and therefore would require less reaming of the anterior cortex. It does, however, violate the elbow capsule. The metaphyseal portal is more proximal and does not violate the capsule. Once the portal is exposed, a guidewire is inserted as careful reaming of the canal is performed so as to ensure minimal stress riser and potential fracture propagation from the portal site. The nail is then inserted with proper visualization of the fracture fragments as well as their reduction, ensuring that the fracture is not nailed in distraction. Locking proximally can be achieved lateral to medial in a freehand manner and is crucial to ensure that the nail does not back out.

C. External Fixation Technique

The placement of the pins depends on the location of the fracture. If proximal pin placement is required, this can be achieved over the lateral surface of the humeral metaphysis, just below the greater trochanter. A distal third fracture may require more distal placement of the proximal pin; this can be achieved on the lateral surface of the shaft. The distal pins can be placed either lateral to medial near the lateral epicondyle or posterior to anterior over the metaphysis. Alternative placement of pins has also been described for very proximal or distal fragments in either the acromion or the ulna, respectively.

The proper placement of the pins when an external fixator is used makes proper visualization of the fracture essential. The patient is placed prone on the table and the fracture is preoperatively visualized with a C arm. This not only ensures proper positioning of the patient but also allows proper positioning of the C arm. The proximal pins may be inserted from lateral to medial with small stab incisions. The incisions are carried to bone and a soft tissue protector is then used to place the pins. Distally, the pins may be placed either lateral to medial or posterior to anterior. If a lateral-to-medial placement is used, the radial nerve may come into play as it courses anterior to posterior. As a result, proper visualization to bone is crucial prior to pin placement. The posterior pins, placed in the midline of the distal third of the humeral shaft, will not threaten any vital structures.

Placement of the connecting bar may be difficult to achieve if the posterior pins are used. In such a case, a small bar may be used to connect the two proximal and two distal pins, followed by a third bar to connect the two bars and stabilize the fracture.

D. Postoperative Care

A sling may be used immediately postoperatively for comfort and to limit initial motion. Range-of-motion exercises should be initiated within a few days with special focus on the finger, wrist and elbow motion. Shoulder exercise institution depends on the stability of the fracture and pain but full shoulder and elbow motion should be obtained by about 1 month postoperatively. Strengthening exercises should be delayed until the fracture is healed.

VIII.   COMPLICATIONS/UNUSUAL CIRCUMSTANCES

A. Gunshot Wounds

Gunshot wounds are a fairly common source of trauma. Humeral shaft fractures occurring as a result of a gunshot wounds are by definition open fractures. In the past, most gunshot wounds were treated with aggressive washout and surgical debridment, not only as a method of preventing infection but also as a means of exploring the extent of the soft tissue injury (46,47). This may have come as a result of studies demonstrating that bullets fired from a gun are not only *not* heat-sterilized but also can draw contaminants such as skin flora or clothing into the wound (48).

More recently, however, some authors are advocating using more conservative management methods, especially with low-velocity (less than 1000ft/s) wounds, as is often seen with civilian firearms. Balfour and Marrero have advocated the use of functional bracing for a specific population of patients with reasonable success. They confined their population to ambulatory patients with midshaft fractures of the humerus who had Gustillo grade II or lower injuries and no associated vascular injury. After initial wound treatment, they applied a modified functional brace and started elbow and shoulder exercise within 1 to 2 weeks of the injury. The time to union was on average 7.5 weeks in patients who cooperated with the rehab program, and the rate of nonunion was just under 2% (16).

Indications for surgical stabilization of fractures caused by gunshot wounds are no different than those for other fractures of the humeral shaft. While most studies include patients with gunshot wounds, no study truly limits its results to these fractures. The use of intramedullary nailing versus plating is again a choice that may be left up to personal preference of the surgeon, depending on the nature of the fracture. In cases where severe soft tissue injury requiring frequent debridment and wound care is present, external fixation has proven to be a good alternative.

B. The Multitrauma Patient

Humeral shaft fractures in multitrauma patients must be addressed in the acute setting in order to minimize associated systemic complications and speed functional recovery. In patient who will need the arm for weight bearing on crutches, intramedullary nailing of the fracture is indicated and has, in one series, led to better rates of union (30). As long as there are no immediate contraindications from one of the associated injuries, stabilizing the fracture in the acute setting may lead to better healing (37).

C. Floating Elbow

The association of humeral shaft fracture with an ipsilateral forearm fracture is seen in sideswipe injuries. In such cases, the outcome of the injury is predicated on the severity of the elbow fracture. Nonunion rates have been reported as high as 100% when these injuries have been treated conservatively (49). Many factors may contribute to this. First, the greater majority of patients suffering from this type of injury are multitrauma patients who may be bedridden. As gravity is an essential component for the success of functional management, be it a hanging arm cast or functional brace, this may contribute to nonunion. In addition, the inherent instability of the fracture pattern may contribute to gross motion at the fracture site and further promote nonunion. As a result, the preferred treatment for these fractures is operative management with either plating or intramedullary rod fixation.

D. Vascular Injury

The presence of a concurrent vascular injury should be carefully evaluated for all humeral shaft fractures. While such injuries are relatively rare, any suspicion of injury should warrant arteriography to determine the indications and site for repair. The presence of a vascular injury can be considered an absolute indication for operative stabilization in order to provide a framework for the vascular repair. Following repair, a fasciotomy of the arm, forearm, and hand may be necessary.

E. Nerve Injury

Due to the course of the radial nerve along the shaft of the humerus, radial nerve palsies are a common occurrence in humeral shaft fracture. The incidence of radial nerve palsies has been reported as high as 15% following humeral shaft fractures (50), with review of the literature indicating an overall rate of about 11% (51). The location of fracture has been a subject of debate as far as direct causality of radial nerve injury. Anatomical studies have demonstrated that the radial nerve may not be in direct contact with the bone in the musculospiral groove, as previously described, but may actually be separated by fibers of the medial head of triceps and brachialis (52). The only time that the nerve was actually in contact with the bone was distally, as it approached the lateral supracondylar ridge. This has brought into question whether the radial nerve is really more at risk with middiaphyseal fractures in comparison with other fracture locations. Several clinical studies have demonstrated a midshaft location as the most common location for associated radial nerve palsies (29,50,53). Pollock et al., however, in a review of 407 consecutive humeral shaft fractures, found that of 24 radial nerve palsies, 15 (63%) were a result of distal fractures (51).

While radial nerve palsies, whether complete or partial, may be a fairly common finding, it has become fairly well established that most do not need exploration and will recover with conservative management. In patients who underwent early exploration of radial nerve palsies, a transected nerve was found in about 12% of cases. In patients who did not undergo exploration, a review indicates that about 73% have spontaneous recovery. In cases when spontaneous recovery did not occur, late exploration revealed a transected nerve in 19% and nerve entrapped in callus in 6% (19,29,50,51,53). In most cases, patients with palsies may be followed closely, with expected recovery (either clinically or through electromyography) by 3 to 4 months. In patients who do not recover by that time, delayed exploration can then be undertaken, with repair in cases where the nerve is lacerated or trapped in callus (51).

F. Pathological Fractures

Pathological fractures are a common finding in orthopedics. The most common malignant neoplasm of bone is metastatic disease. While the most common site for metastatic disease is the femur, the humerus is next commonly affected, with as many as 16% of 588 pathological fractures in one series (54). Most of these fractures are associated with severe pain and a loss of function in the affected extremity. The most common primary site is breast, with one series quoting an 18.6% of 103 breast cancer patients developing humeral shaft metastasis (55).

Unlike regular fractures of the humeral shaft, pathological fractures usually do not achieve good results when treated conservatively (55). As a result, most authors will agree that surgical stabilization of the fracture is important for achieving functional use of the affected extremity and adequate pain control. These factors may be crucial in improving the quality of life of these patients as well as reducing the need for nursing and assisted living situations.

IX. CONCLUSION

Fractures of the humeral shaft are fairly common injuries. The surrounding anatomy of the humeral shaft and the presence of gravity make it unique in that most fractures can be successfully treated nonoperatively with functional bracing, with excellent results. In cases where surgery is indicated, the option of plating versus intramedullary nailing provides the surgeon with multiple options for fixation, depending on the characteristics of the fracture and any associated diseases or fractures. In cases of severely comminuted fractures, external fixation of the fracture is an alternative method. Outcomes are favorable in most cases regardless of the method of fixation as long as special care is taken in the postoperative period to ensure proper restoration of range of motion and function of the shoulder and elbow.

REFERENCES

1. EF Ward, FH Savoie III, JL Hughes. Fractures of the diaphyseal humerus. In: Browner BD, Levine AM, Trafton PG, eds. *Skeletal Trauma*. Philadelphia: Saunders, 1998, pp 1523–1547.
2. J Caldwell. Treatment of fractures of the shaft of the humerus by hanging cast. *Surg Gynecol Obstet* 70:421–425, 1940.
3. C Holm. Management of humeral shaft fractures—Fundamental nonoperative technics. *Clin Orthop Rel Res* 71:132–139, 1970.
4. A Sarmiento, PB Kinman, EG Galvin, RH Schmitt, JG Phillips. Functional bracing of fractures of the humerus. *J Bone Joint Surg* 59A(5):596–601, 1977.
5. H Gray. Osteology—The appendicular skeleton. In: Clemente C, ed. Anatomy of the Human Body. Baltimore: Williams & Wilkins, 1985, ch. 4.
6. S Carroll. A study of the nutrient foramina of the humeral diaphysis. *J Bone Joint Surg* 45B(1):176–181, 1963.
7. S Hoppenfield, P deBoer. Surgical Exposures in Orthopaedics—The Anatomic Approach. Philadelphia: Lippincott, 1984, ch. 2.
8. L Klenerman. Experimental fractures of the adult humerus. *Med Biol Eng* 7:357–364, 1969.
9. CG Finkemeier. RR Slater, Jr. Fractures and dislocations of the shoulder girdle and humerus. In: MW Chapman, ed. *Chapman's Orthopaedic Surgery*. Philadelphia: Lippincott Williams & Wilkins, 2001, pp 463–480.
10. T Ruedi, L Schweiberer. Scapula, clavicle, humerus. In: Muller ME, Schneider R, eds. *Manual of Internal Fixation: Techniques Recommended by the AO-ASIF Group*. Berlin: Springer-Verlag, 1991, pp 427–452.
11. RB Gustilo, JT Anderson. Prevention of infection in the treatment of one thousand and twenty-five open fractures of long bones. *J Bone Joint Surg* 58A(4):453–458, 1976.
12. PR Gregory, Jr. Fractures of the shaft of the humerus. In: Buscholz RW, ed. *Rockwood and Green's Fractures in Adults*. Philadelphia: Lippincott/William & Wilkins, 2001, pp 973–996, ch. 24.
13. GW Balfour, V Mooney, ME Ashby. Diaphyseal fractures of the humerus treated with a ready-made fracture brace. *J Bone Joint Surg* 64A(1):11–13, 1982.
14. A Sarmiento, JP Waddell, LL Latta. Diaphyseal humeral fractures: Treatment options. *AAOS Instr Course Lect* 51:257–278, 2002.
15. JB Zagorski, LL Latta, GA Zych, AR Finnieston. Diaphyseal fractures of the humerus—Treatment with prefabricated braces. *J Bone Joint Surg* 70A(4):607–610, 1988.
16. GW Balfour, CE Marrero. Fracture brace for the treatment of humerus shaft fractures caused by gunshot wounds. *Orthop Clin North Am* 26(1):55–63, 1995.
17. D Heim, F Herbert, P Hess, P Regazzoni. Surgical treatment of humeral shaft fractures—The Basel experience. *J Trauma*, 35(2):226–232, 1993.
18. RM Pickering, AH Crenshaw, Jr., DM Zinar. Intramedullary nailing of humeral shaft fractures. *AAOS Instr Course Lect* 51:271–278, 2002.

19. L Klenerman. Fractures of the shaft of the humerus. *J Bone Joint Surg* 48B(1): 105–111, 1966.

20. EJ Dabezies, CJ Banta II, CP Murphy, RD d'Ambrosia. Plate fixation of the humeral shaft for acute fractures, with and without radial nerve injuries. *J Orthop Trauma* 6(1):10–13, 1992.

21. MJ Bell, CJ Beauchamp, JK Kellam, RY McMurtry. The results of plating humeral shaft fractures in patients with multiple injuries—The Sunnybrook experience. *J Bone Joint Surg* 67B:293–296, 1985.

22. JR Chapman, MB Henley, J Agel, PJ Benca. Randomized prospective study of humeral shaft fractures: Intramedullary nails versus plates. *J Orthop Trauma* 14(3): 162–166, 2000.

23. RJ Foster, GL Dixon, AW Bach, RW Appleyard, TM Green. Internal fixation of fractures and non-union of the humeral shaft. *J Bone Joint Surg* 67A(6):857–864, 1985.

24. J Lin. Treatment of humeral shaft fractures with humeral locked nail and comparison with plate fixation. *J Trauma* 44(5):859–864, 1998.

25. PJ O'Brien, G. Pierre, PA Blachut. Humeral shaft fractures: Open reduction internal fixation. In: DA Wiss, ed. *Master Techniques in Orthopaedic Surgery*. Philadelphia: Lippincott-Raven, 1998, pp 63–79.

26. P Laing. The arterial supply of the adult humerus. *J Bone Joint Surg* 38A(5): 1105–1116, 1956.

27. J Crates. AP Whittle. Antegrade interlocking nailing of acute humeral shaft fractures. *Clin Orthop Rel Res* 350:40–50, 1998.

28. WA Bleeker, NW Nijsten, HJT Duis. Treatment of humeral shaft fractures related to associated injuries. *Acta Orthop Scand* 62(2):148–153, 1991.

29. JW Mast, PG Spiegel, JP Harvey, C Harrison. Fractures of the humeral shaft—A retrospective study of 240 adult fractures. *Clin Orthop Rel Res* 112:254–262, 1975.

30. R Vander Griend, J Tomasin, EF Ward. Open reduction and internal fixation of humeral shaft fractures—Results using AO plating techniques. *J Bone Joint Surg* 68A(3):430–433, 1986.

31. RA Durbin, MJ Gottesman, KC Sanders. Hackethal stacked nailing of humeral shaft fractures: Experiences with 30 patients. *Clin Orthop Rel Res* 179:168–174, 1983.

32. B Riemer. Humeral shaft fractures: Intramedulalry nailing. In: DA Wiss, ed. *Master Techniques in Orthopaedic Surgery*. Philadelphia: Lippincott-Raven, 1998, pp 81–94.

33. D Strothman, DC Templeman, T Varecka, J Bechtold. Retrograde nailing of humeral shaft fractures: A biomechanical study of its effects on the strength of the distal humerus. *J Orthop Trauma* 14(2):101–104, 2000.

34. BL Riemer, SL Butterfield, R D'Ambrosia, J Kellam. Seidel intramedullary nailing of humeral diaphyseal fractures: A preliminary report. *Orthopaedics* 14:239–246, 1991.

35. J Lin, SM Hou, YS Hang, EYS Chao. Treatment of humeral shaft fractures by retrograde locked nailing. *Clin Orthop Rel Res* 342:147–155, 1997.

36. PM Rommens, J Blum, M Runkel. Retrograde nailing of humeral shaft fractures. *Clin Orthop Rel Res* 350:26–39, 1998.

37. RJ Brumback, MJ Bosse, A Poka, AR Burgess. Intramedullary stabilization of humeral shaft fractures in patients with multiple trauma. *J Bone Joint Surg* 68A: 960–970, 1986.

38. J Crates. AP Whittle. Antegrade interlocking nailing of acute humeral shaft fractures. *Clin Orthop Rel Res* 350:40–50, 1998.

39. PJ Stern, DL Mattingly, DL Pomeroy, EJ Zenni, JK Kreig. Intramedullary fixation of humeral shaft fractures. *J Bone Joint Surg* 66A(5):639–646, 1984.

40. CM Robinson, KM Bell, CM Court-Brown, MM McQueen. Locked nailing of humeral shaft fractures—Experience in Edinburgh over a 2-year period. *J Bone Joint Surg* 74B:558–562, 1992.

41. MA Cox, M Dolan, K Synnott, JP McElwain. Closed interlocking nailing of humeral shaft fractures with the Russell-Taylor nail. *J Orthop Trauma* 14(5):349–353, 2000.

42. AM Ingman, DA Waters. Locked intramedullary nailing of humeral shaft fractures: Implant design, surgical technique and clinical results. *J Bone Joint Surg* 76B:23–29, 1994.

43. JB Rathbun, I Macnab. The Microvascular pattern of the rotator cuff. *J Bone Joint Surg* 52B(3):540–553, 1970.

44. HR Mostafavi, P Tornetta III. Open fractures of the humeral shaft treated with external fixation. *Clin Orthop Rel Res* 337:187–197, 1997.

45. TF Wisniewski, MJ Radziejowski. Gunshot fractures of the humeral shaft treated with external fixation. *J Orthop Trauma* 10(4):273–278, 1996.

46. J Trueta. Treatment of war fractures by the closed method. *Lancet* 1:1173, 1937.

47. H Ziperman. The management of soft-tissue missile wounds in war and peace. *J Trauma* 1:361, 1961.

48. FP Thoresby, HM Darlow. The mechanism of primary infection of bullet wounds. *J Bone Joint Surg* 54A:359, 1967.

49. RH Lange, RJ Foster. Skeletal management of humeral shaft fractures associated with forearm fractures. *Clin Orthop Rel Res* 195:173–177, 1985.

50. DB Kettelkamp, HH Alexander. Clinical review of radial nerve injury. *J Trauma* 7:424–432, 1967.

51. FH Pollock, D Drake, EG Bovill, L Day, PG Trafton. Treatment of radial neuropathy associated with fractures of the humerus. *J Bone Joint Surg* 63A(2):239–243, 1981.

52. R Whitson. Relation of the radial nerve to the shaft of the humerus. *J Bone Joint Surg* 36A:85–88, 1954.

53. A Garcia, BH Maeck. Radial nerve injuries in fractures of the shaft of the humerus. *Am J Surg* 99:625–627, 1960.

54. ET Habermann, RA Lopez. Metastatic disease of bone and treatment of pathological fractures. *Orthop Clin North Am* 20:469–486, 1989.

55. JE Flemming, RK Beabi. Pathologic fracture of the humerus. *Clin Orthop Rel Res* 203:258–260, 1986.

6

Nonunions of the Upper Extremity

Wade R. Smith, Ian Pallister, and Kirti Moholkar
Denver Health Medical Center, Denver, Colorado, U.S.A.

Advancements in fracture care have significantly improved the outcome of upper extremity injuries. However, nonunions continue to occur, often with devastating functional sequelae. Improvements in patient resuscitation, car safety, and surgical technology have changed the nature of upper extremity nonunions. Before the era of airbags, lowered speed limits, trauma systems, and open reduction techniques, nonunions occurred primarily in low-energy injuries treated by nonoperative methods. When healing did not occur, the result was often a hypertrophic nonunion. In current practice, hypertrophic nonunions continue to be seen, but an increasing percentage of nonunions are atrophic and infected and may be complicated by significant bone loss, soft tissue deficits and nerve damage. The complex reconstructive processes required for subsequent treatment have complications of their own, including reflex sympathetic dystrophy, disabling sensory or motor function of the extremity, and permanent functional impairment. In order to avoid complications and ensure the best possible outcome in each individual case, a systematic evaluation of the etiology and type of nonunion must be undertaken. Additionally, the patient must be carefully evaluated psychosocially so that the treating physician understands the patient's capacity for various treatments as well as his or her expectations and the level of function the patient requires to resume normal activities. The surgeon should be facile with a variety of approaches to the problem and be capable of educating the patient as to the efficacy and potential risk/benefit of each approach. When all of these conditions are satisfied, the patient and surgeon together have the greatest chance of choosing a treatment path that will avoid the pitfalls and ultimately result in a healed fracture with maximal preservation of function.

I. EVALUATION

Evaluation and diagnosis of an upper extremity nonunion can be difficult because of the non-weight-bearing nature of the involved structures. However, if
an accurate diagnosis is not formed—which must include the etiology and type
of nonunion as well as systemic and patient-related factors—an optimal treatment plan cannot be reliably accomplished. Initial evaluation should account for
the mechanism and severity of the initial injury: Was this a high- or low-energy
injury? Was the fracture open or closed? Were there other associated injuries of
the head, chest, abdomen, or musculoskeletal system? How many and what type
of operations were performed? Were there any complications, such as nerve injuries? The history should also provide a picture of the postinjury course and the
goals of the patient: What type of residual physical and mental disabilities are
present? Did the patient attend physical therapy? Is the patient a tobacco user?
Are there other substance abuse issues? What type of work does the patient
perform now, if any, and to what type of work does he or she expect to return?
Last, the primary complaint must be reconciled with the preceding information:
Is the degree of pain and disability significantly affecting the patient's life? The
presence of a nonunion on x-ray does not necessarily require intervention if the
risk/benefit ratio is not in the patient's favor. In some cases of severely disabled
polytrauma or life-threatening medical conditions, though rare, surgical intervention for an upper extremity nonunion is not in the patient's best interest.

   The physical examination should focus on the presence or absence of pain
at the nonunion site, range of motion of the adjacent joints, and an accurate
neurovascular examination of the extremity. Evidence of previous scars, surgical
incisions, or draining sinuses should be noted and documented. Length of the
limb and rotational or angular deformity should be compared to the other side,
although these indices are less critical in the upper extremity than in the lower
limbs. The motor examination should attempt to differentiate between decreased
strength from disuse versus nerve or muscle damage. The examiner must be
careful to prove that pain is from the suspected nonunion site and not from an
ipsilateral injury, such as a rotator cuff tear, or from a chronic pain syndrome,
such as reflex sympathetic dystrophy, neuroma, or cervical spine lesion.

   A careful history and physical examination will lead to a thorough imaging
examination. High-quality orthogonal x-rays of the extremity, which include the
adjacent joints, are mandatory. If possible, comparison to the original treatment
films will facilitate diagnosis. In cases of fracture gap, bone loss, or hardware
failure, the diagnosis may be obvious. In other cases, the presence and type of
nonunion will remain unclear and further imaging will be required. Oblique
views, tomograms, technetium bone scans and computed tomography can eluci-
date the presence and extent of a nonunion as well as delineate the amount of
callus or bone present. Indium white blood cell scans and MRI provide information regarding the presence and extent of infection. Laboratory values including
white blood cell count, erythrocyte sedimentation rate (ESR), and C-reactive
protein (CRP) should be obtained in every evaluation of nonunion.

The end result of the evaluation process should be a diagnosis that includes the presence or absence of nonunion, the type of nonunion (atrophic, hypertrophic, or infected), and the cause(s) of the problem. A clear picture should be formed of the patient, the problem, and specific challenges to successful treatment, such as dense scars, disability, or smoking. At this point, a preoperative plan must be devised.

II. PREOPERATIVE PLANNING

Once the decision to proceed with surgery has been made, the type of surgery best suited to the patient and the situation must be chosen. Regardless of technique, the basic elements of preoperative planning consist of preparation and education of both the patient and the surgical team. The patient must clearly understand the treatment and what will be required in the postoperative period in terms of physical therapy, limb lengthening, and pain control. Whenever possible, a preoperative physical therapy assessment can provide a baseline while also teaching the patient about initial treatment. Comorbidities necessitate preoperative medical evaluation. Plastic or vascular surgery consultation should be considered in the case of compromised skin or blood supply. The health and fitness of the patient for the proposed surgery should not be neglected in any respect for the sake of expediency.

Surgical preparation requires templating of the nonunion. There are several useful techniques, but the simplest is to trace the united or malunited fragments with tracing paper held over the relevant radiographs (1). These fragments are then cut out and taped into appropriate alignment. Implant templates can then be placed under the tracing paper and drawings made to allow preplanning of the implant, its size, the number and size of screws, or position and type of wires. Length and width of intramedullary nails can be estimated from anteroposterior (AP) and lateral radiographs with 10 to 15% subtraction for magnification. Limb-lengthening or bone-transport goals should be determined by clinical examination and accounted for in the preoperative plan. The need for bone grafting should be predetermined, as well as the type and site of the graft.

The preoperative plan must account for all implants to be extracted or implanted. Appropriate extraction tools should be ordered so that they will be available in the operating room as needed. Some type of broken screw or rod removal set should be available. Special considerations—such as radiolucent tables, fluoroscopy, intraoperative Gram stains, or frozen tissue sections—should be in the plan. Communication with the surgical staff to ensure appropriate assistance and familiarity with the planned operation are imperative. It is the surgeon's responsibility to ensure that the operative staff is properly educated and prepared for the procedure.

When preoperative planning is completed, the surgical team should know exactly what they will do and that all the necessary components will be present in the operating room. If the plan is incomplete or in doubt, the surgery should be delayed until all issues are resolved. Nonunion surgery in the upper extremity is fraught with potential complications, which can be avoided by proper planning. The surgeon should consider the proposed procedure in the same light as an expedition to the top of Mt. Everest: proper planning prevents poor performance.

III.   NONUNION OF THE HUMERUS

A high percentage of humeral diaphyseal fractures heal with nonoperative treatment. Whether surgical intervention is chosen or not, union rates approach 95% (2). When nonunion does occur after nonoperative treatment, likely causes include a high level of severity of the initial injury, distraction of the fracture, soft tissue damage or interposition, transverse or short oblique fracture patterns, and/ or inadequate immobilization (3–6). Smoking, alcoholism, obesity, and the type of nonoperative treatment can be secondary contributory factors. In cases of nonunion following nonoperative treatment, compression or wave plating, intramedullary reamed nailing and external fixation have all proven to be effective treatment modalities (7–10).

Nonunion following primary surgical treatment can be caused by inadequate stabilization, distraction or lack of contact of the bone ends, osteopenia, infection, lack of blood supply, or soft tissue inadequacy. Like nonoperative nonunions, comorbidities can significantly retard bone healing. Operative treatment choices may be more complex because of bone loss, soft tissue defects, or the presence of infection. In both operative and nonoperative nonunions, adjunctive bone graft is desirable in specific subsets of patients but is not required in all (9,11).

A.   Operative Techniques in Humeral Shaft Nonunions

Preoperative evaluation and planning allow the surgeon to make a precise diagnosis and determine the type of nonunion. Subsequent surgical treatment should thus fit the problem and not be limited to a single technique. Surgeons dealing with nonunion must become facile with a variety of operative approaches and solutions. Understandably, each surgeon will feel that specific techniques are better than others. However, to be limited to one technique only is to limit the patient's chances of a successful outcome. Therefore, in examining operative technique, a problem-focused approach is useful.

B.   Hypertrophic Nonunions

The hallmark of a hypertrophic nonunion is abundant callus formation without complete healing. In the humerus, these calluses are often the result of failed nonoperative treatment or operative intervention without adequate mechanical stability. A healthy vascular environment allows callus formation, but lack of appropriate stability prevents complete maturation and healing of calluses. Thus the problem is lack of stability and the solution is to provide stability while preserving vascular supply to the fracture site (Fig. 1). Surgical options include open reduction internal fixation (ORIF) with compression, reamed intramedul-

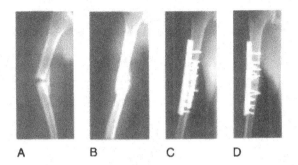

Figure 1 Hypertrophic nonunion of the humeral shaft. A. Preoperative AP view after 9 months of cast brace treatment. B. Preoperative lateral view. C. Postoperative AP view following compression plating with anterior tension-band plate. D. Postoperative lateral view.

lary nailing, and external fixation with monolateral or ring fixators. Bone graft has not been shown to be necessary if appropriate stability and compression is provided at the fracture site (7,11).

C. Atrophic Nonunion

Atrophic nonunions lack callus formation and may exhibit bone resorption at the fracture site. The etiology is biological, representing a failure of fracture hematoma to transform into callus. Gross instability, severe soft tissue injury, and infection predispose to atrophic nonunion. In uninfected cases, stable fixation with minimal disruption of the surrounding blood supply is necessary as well as adjunctive bone grafting. The osteoprogenitor cells and osteoinductive and conductive components provided in bone graft aid the deficient biological environment and promote resumption of bone synthesis.

Compression at the fracture site is not always achievable because of bony defects. Consequently, the implant construct in atrophic nonunions must be able to withstand potentially longer periods until fracture union, and inadequate fixation is more susceptible to failure. Alternatively, bone gaps can be bridged by vascularized or tricortical grafts, which allow for cortical bone on bone contact at the fracture site and increase the construct's stability. Shortening of 2 to 3 cm in the humerus also allows for bone-on-bone compression and increases fixation stability. Wave plate fixation, reamed intramedullary nailing, compression plating, and distraction osteogenesis with the Ilizarov apparatus have all been described as effective treatments in atrophic nonunion of the humerus.

D. Infection

Infected humeral fractures result after open injury or after surgical repair. The rate of infection after ORIF has been reported as at 0 to 5% (3–6,11). Infected nonunions are usually atrophic and represent a management challenge. The first step is to diagnose the infection. All nonunions must include a thorough evaluation to exclude infection prior to definitive treatment. After diagnosis, the extent of infection must be determined. Magnetic resonance imaging (MRI) has become an effective tool in estimating the longitudinal extent of osteomyelitis in long bones, but it can be overread, leading to excessive bone debridement. Indium-labeled white blood cell scans can aid in differentiating infection from aseptic nonunion. There is controversy regarding the need for total versus subtotal debridement of osteomyelitis, and there are no specific data for the humerus. Our practice is to estimate the extent of osteomyelitis from a combination of imaging studies, depending upon the duration, magnitude, and clinical symptomatology of the lesion. Bone resection should be part of the preoperative plan, so that contingencies can be planned for, with appropriate fixation available as well as void fillers such as antibiotic-impregnated beads. Three general approaches in the humerus are as follows: (1) bone debridement with subsequent internal fixation with either a plate or nail construct (12), (2) ring fixator application with either acute shortening or distraction osteogenesis (7,13), and (3) temporary monolateral external fixation with staged grafting and internal fixation or intramedullary nailing (12,14). Soft tissue coverage may be required, as well as prolonged administration of intravenous antibiotics.

E. Open Reduction with Internal Fixation

Open reduction techniques for humeral nonunion are well described, with reported union rates ranging from 80 to 96% (3–6,11). Jupiter specifically described treatment of atrophic nonunion in obese patients with a medial approach, anterior plate, and vascularized fibular graft. All four nonunions that were treated healed, but not without complication (9). Radial nerve palsy remains a potential risk and is reported to occur in 3 to 29% of nonunion cases (14). The principles of successful treatment include protecting the radial nerve, resecting atrophic nonunions, shortening as required to achieve apposition of well-vascularized fragments, use of a dynamic compression plate, achieving compression at the fracture site, and grafting with cancellous bone (11) (Fig. 2).

Three standard approaches are preferred: anterolateral (15), direct lateral (16), and direct posterior (15). The choice of approach is predicated upon several factors, including the presence of scars from previous surgery, location of the nonunion, presence of radial nerve injury, and health status of the patient. The anterolateral and lateral approaches allow supine positioning, while the posterior approach requires the patient to be either in the lateral decubitus position or prone. The anterolateral and direct lateral approaches allow for extensile exposure of the humerus. Both permit isolation and examination of the radial nerve; however, the direct lateral provides the most extensile exposure of the radial nerve proximally. The posterior approach avoids the radial nerve in the distal third of the humerus, but the nerve directly crosses the operative field in the middle third (17).

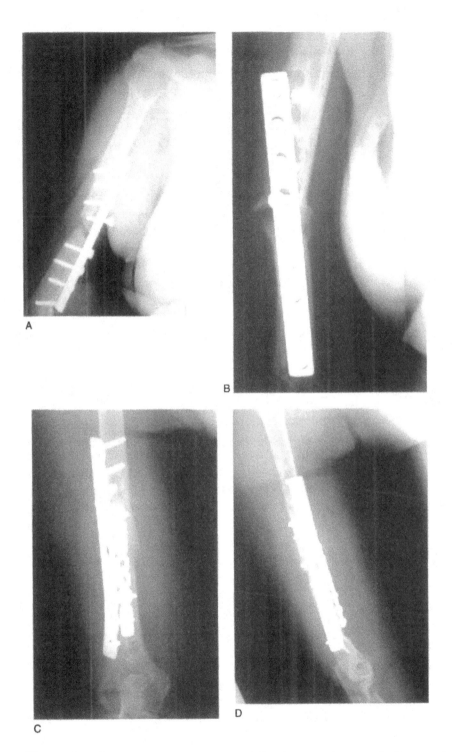

Figure 2 Atropic nonunion of humerus following open fracture. A. Preoperative anteroposterior (AP) view. B. AP view of anterior plate with implant failure and angulation. C. Postoperative AP view 3 months following compression plating with demineralized bone matrix graft. D. Postoperative lateral view with cortical bridging in both planes.

If the radial nerve is in the field during the surgical approach, it should be identified and carefully protected. A wide vessel loop or narrow Penrose drain is placed to protect the nerve. Thin vessel loops have a tendency to pull tightly through a small area and may cause more damage to the nerve. The humerus and previously placed implants should be identified. At this juncture it is critical that only enough periosteal dissection be performed to permit implant removal. In hypertrophic nonunions, it is not necessary to take down the entire nonunion. The goal is to stabilize the nonunion site by improving the mechanics of the fixation. In cases with abundant hypertrophic callus, a single narrow 4.5-mm dynamic compression plate is sufficient as long as compression is achieved either through the plate's compression holes or outside the plate with an external tensioning device. The length of the plate is determined from the preoperative template. A minimum of six cortices should be fixed with bicortical screws on either side of the nonunion. When a plate is removed, the new plate should span past the original screw holes at each end. In these cases or when the nonunion site spans several centimeters, eight cortices of fixation on either side should be achieved. When the fracture gap appears to be greater than 3 to 5 mm between the bone ends, the external tensioner or other technique, such as use of a laminar spreader positioned against the plate and a screw outside the plate, should be used to reduce the gap. Theoretically, compression through the plate permits 1 mm of compression per hole, and it is usually difficult to achieve more than 3 mm of total compression solely through the plate. A small amount of callus may be removed to allow better contact between the plate and the bone. It is of utmost importance that compression of the bone ends be achieved, as this provides most of the increased stability required to transform a hypertrophic nonunion into a healed fracture. On the table, radiographs are taken to confirm that the preoperative goals were achieved and then a layered closure is performed. Physical therapy should begin as soon as possible, with an emphasis on range of motion of the shoulder and elbow. If the surgical goals are met, prognosis is excellent for eventual union.

F. Intramedullary Nailing

Intramedullary nailing of humeral nonunions using a variety of implants has been described (8,10,12,14,18–21). However, there is a relative paucity of reports regarding the current generation of intramedullary implants (Fig. 3). The most effective technique appears to be statically locked humeral nails with open bone grafting. In regard to the efficacy of bone healing, there is no significant difference between a retrograde and an antegrade approach. In their series, Lin et al. (14) reported a 94.1% healing rate, with a mean time to union of 5.6 months. They advocated open bone grafting, static locking, and careful exposure of the radial nerve. Earlier reports with nonlocking nails yielded poorer results (16,22,23). Exchange nailing of previously nailed nonunions resulted in less than a 50% union rate, despite reaming and placement of large-diameter nails (12). It

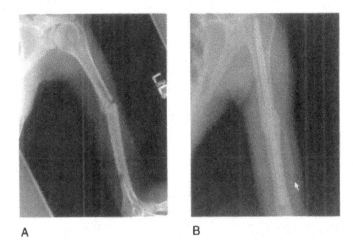

A   B

Figure 3   Hypertophic nonunion treated with inflatable intramedullary nail. A. Preoperative view. B. Postoperative AP view with callus at 3 months. (Courtesy of Bruce Ziran, M.D., University of Pittsburgh Medical Center, Pittsburgh, Pennsylvania.)

is unknown whether reaming aids or hinders healing of humeral nonunions. The presumed role of reaming has been extrapolated from experience in nonunion treatment of the lower extremity. Likewise, differences between antegrade and retrograde humeral nailing have not been well elucidated (24). The principal goals of intramedullary nailing are precisely the same as those of compression plating: bony stability, maintenance of soft tissue viability, and early functional rehabilitation. Intramedullary nailing of the humerus can be technically demanding, whether in the treatment of acute or ununited fractures. Problems to consider prior to surgery are potential complications related to shoulder or elbow function, the feasibility of obtaining compression at the fracture site, and the potential for radial nerve injury if a closed technique is selected. Additional barriers to a successful outcome include difficulties in imaging and positioning. While intramedullary nailing of humeral nonunions appears conceptually to be a simpler and less invasive procedure, it may in fact make it more difficult to achieve stability and be more dangerous to neurovascular structures, depending on the experience of the surgeon. Current studies focusing on nonlocked expandable stainless steel nails and combinations of intramedullary nailing with simultaneous external fixation may expand the role of nailing in humeral nonunions.

G.   Ilizarov Ring Fixation

Circular ring fixation provides an alternative method for applying compression and stability to a hypertrophic nonunion. Numerous authors have described successful results with the use of the Ilizarov fixator (7,13,19,25–27) (Fig. 4). Patel et al. treated 16 humeral nonunions with Ilizarov ring fixation (27). Ten nonunions followed intramedullary nailing and were successfully treated in a closed

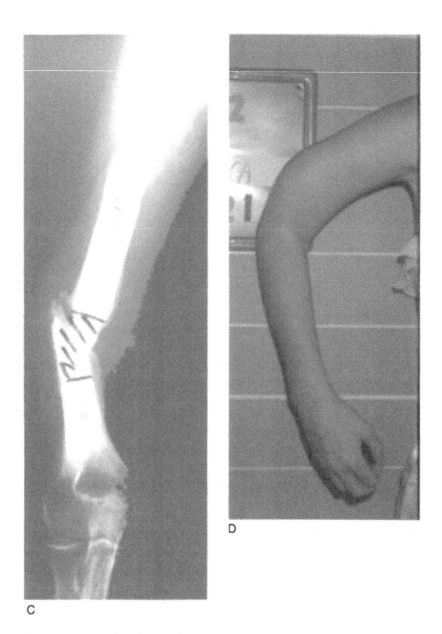

C

D

Figure 3 Continued. C. Postoperative view following intramedullary nail. D. Postoperative view following debridement and nail extraction. (Courtesy of Maurizio Catagni, M.D., Ospedale de Lecco, Lecco, Italy.)

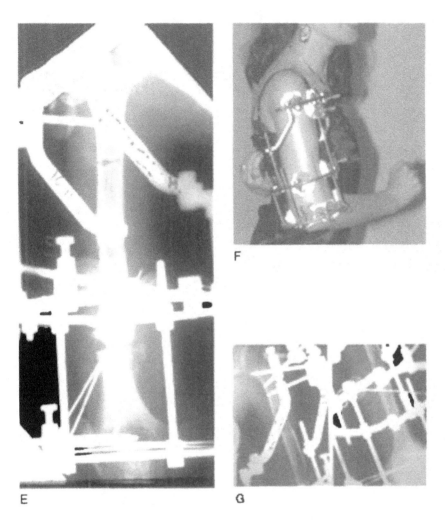

E   G

Figure 3 Continued.   E. Clinical appearance of right arm with nonunion. F. Postoperative AP view following bone resection and Ilizarov placement with corticotomy.
G. Postoperative view of patient with full range of motion, with 90 degree range of
motion of the elbow. (Courtesy of Maurizio Catagni, M.D., Ospedale de Lecco, Lecco,
Italy.)

fashion by using the ring fixator to compress the bone ends over the retained
nail. Of 6 remaining nonunions, 5 achieved healing after implant removal, debridement, and compression. Bone grafting was not used. There were no deep
infections, but three nerve injuries resulted, all of which resolved within 3
months. Lammens et al. (13) used monofocal compression in 30 humeri; 14
nonunions were hypertrophic and 16 were atrophic, with 6 infections. Of the 30
humeri, 28 achieved union without additional bone grafting. There were no nerve
injuries or deep infections.

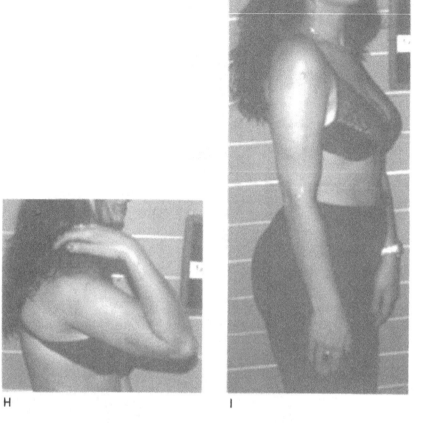

H   I

Figure 3 Continued. H and I. Extension and flexion of the elbow following removal of Ilizarov frame and healing of fracture and infection. (Courtesy of Maurizio Catagni, M.D., Ospedale de Lecco, Lecco, Italy.

1. Technique

The patient can be placed supine or lying in a beach chair. Previously placed hardware should be removed through a standard approach based on the original surgery. In the case of aseptic nonunion with an intramedullary nail, distal interlocks can be removed to facilitate compression at the nonunion site. In hypertrophic nonunions, the fracture site is not debrided. In atrophic nonunions, dead bone is debrided until there is bleeding bone at both ends. Bone graft can be added if there is absolute certainty that the nonunion is aseptic. Infected nonunions are aggressively debrided, and antibiotic beads can be added. A resulting bone gap of up to 3 cm may be acutely compressed to avoid the need for bone transport. If a larger bone deficit is present after debridement, a distant corticotomy should be added to permit distraction osteogenesis. A standard construct would include a minimum of a five-eighths ring at the elbow, a full ring at the

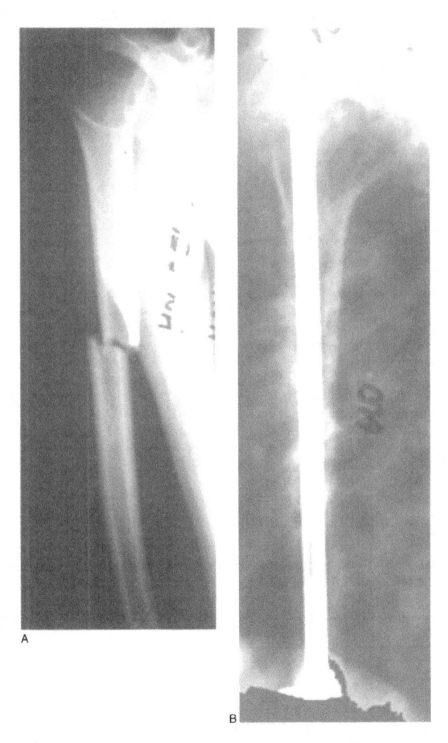

Figure 4 Atropic nonunion of humerus following intramedullary nailing treated with Ilizarov ring fixation. A and B. AP and lateral preoperative views. (Courtesy of Maurizio Catagni, M.D., Ospedale de Lecco, Lecco, Italy.)

middiaphysis, and one to two partial arches proximally. We prefer the hybrid advanced technique as described by Catagni (7), which employs a combination of thin wires and half pins (Fig. 5) Compression is achieved after frame placement. Care must be taken to make sure that the frame allows full range of motion at the elbow and shoulder and that it will not impinge on the chest when the arm is normally positioned. We begin immediate range-of-motion exercises, permit use of the arm for activities of daily living, and, if necessary, permit weight bearing with crutches or a walker.

H. Summary

Nonunions of the humerus should be approached in a systematic manner so that appropriate treatment can be planned. The nature and cause of the nonunion must be determined by a thorough history and physical examination combined with appropriate laboratory and imaging modalities. Hypertrophic nonunions can be effectively treated with ORIF, reamed intramedullary nailing, or monofocal Ilizarov ring fixation (Fig. 6). Atrophic nonunions require stabilization and bone grafting or bone transport (Fig. 7). Vascularized grafts have been reported, but the indications in the humerus are not well elucidated. Infected nonunions can be treated by a staged protocol including bone debridement, antibiotic bead placement, temporary external fixation, and subsequent ORIF with bone grafting or by a single-stage protocol employing either monolateral external fixation or Ilizarov treatment with distraction osteogenesis. Each of these treatments requires specific expertise and experience. Whichever modality is chosen, the surgeon must be aware of the increased risk of complications, including infection, iatrogenic nerve injury, and functional disability of the extremity (Fig. 8). Preoperative planning can decrease complication rates and permit a better surgical and functional outcome.

IV. NONUNIONS OF THE ELBOW

Fractures about the elbow are relatively uncommon, and problems of nonunion can largely be avoided by optimum primary treatment. However, nonunions do occur and, in the case of fractures of the distal humerus, have an incidence of approximately 3 to 5% (25). They are twice as common in females, especially

---

FACING PAGE

Figure 4   Infected nonunion of the forearm following open reduction internal fixation. C and D. AP and lateral views at presentation, showing hardware failure and 1-year nonunion. E. Initial postoperative view after implant removable bone resection, corticotomy, and transport of the ulna. F. Postoperative view after 4 cm of ulnar transport and docking. Patient had functional wrist and elbow motion after complete healing and therapy. (Courtesy of Maurizio Catagni, M.D., Ospedale de Lecco, Lecco, Italy.)

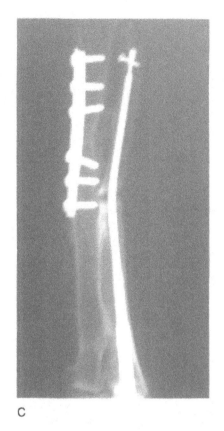

C

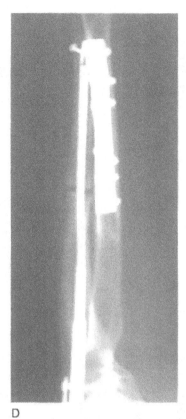

D

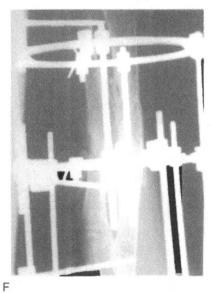

E

F

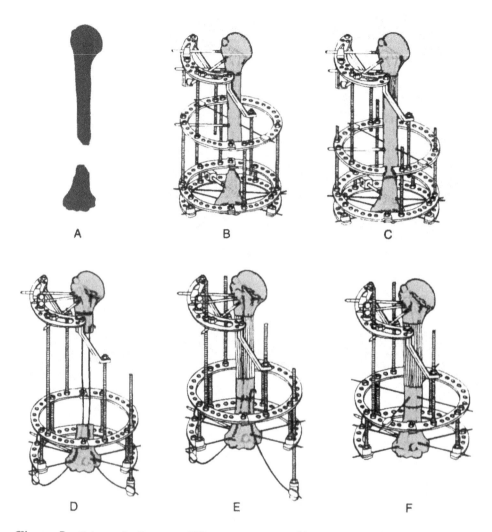

Figure 5 Schematic diagram of Ilizarov treatment of humeral nonunion. A to C. Treatment of bone defect with hybrid advanced frame and distraction osteogenesis. D to F. Treatment of a massive defect with "pull wire" technique and distraction osteogenesis. (Courtesy of Maurizio Catagni, M.D., Ospedale de Lecco, Lecco, Italy.)

the elderly (26). Factors in the development of nonunion may be related to the original injury itself, the patient, and the initial treatment adopted.

The location of the injury, the integrity of the overlying soft tissues, and fracture type are important considerations. High-energy patterns of injury will result in fracture comminution, damage to the soft tissue envelope, and possibly devascularization of bony fragments. Distal humeral fractures in particular are relatively common in the elderly, in whom a degree of osteoporosis is invariably present. Iatrogenic factors center on failure to achieve adequate stabilization of

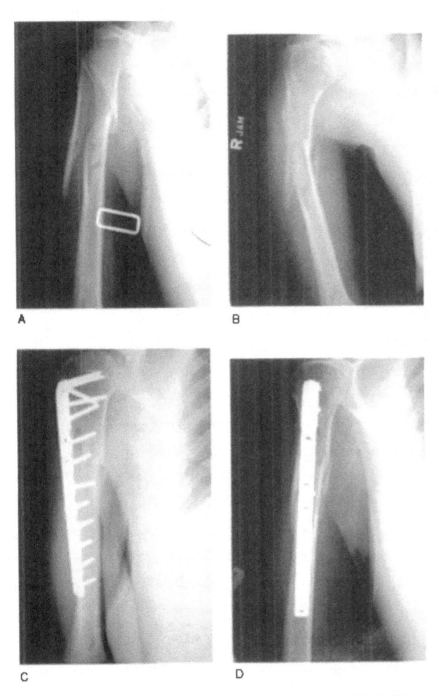

Figure 6 Proximal third humeral shaft nonunion treated initially without surgery. A and B. Preoperative AP and lateral views 6 months after injury, showing minimal callus. C and D. Postoperative views showing early healing at 2 months. (Courtesy of Steven J. Morgan, M.D., Denver Health Medical Center, Denver, Colorado.)

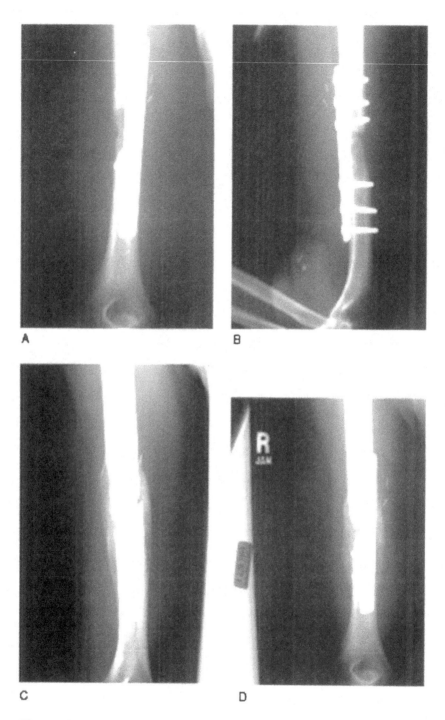

Figure 7 Atrophic humeral nonunion treated with bone grafting. A. Preoperative AP view showing lack of callus. B. Preoperative lateral view. C. Postoperative AP view after 3 months, with new callus formation. Original hardware was retained and only autograft bone was added to the nonunion site. D. Lateral view with healing. (Courtesy of Steven J. Morgan, M.D., Denver Health Medical Center, Denver, Colorado.)

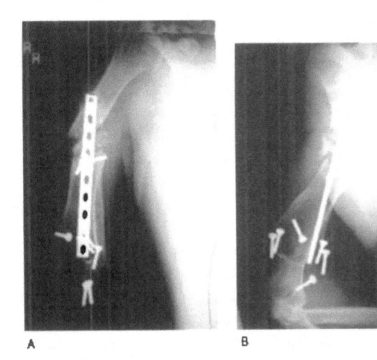

A   B

Figure 8 Humeral nonunion with hardware failure. The patient had multiple medial contraindications to surgery, including Childs C liver disease, and chose nonoperative care, as he was only moderately symptomatic. (Courtesy of Steven J. Morgan, M.D., Denver Health Medical Center, Denver, Colorado.)

the fracture fragments, sometimes complicated by the introduction of infection at the time of surgery.

The treatment goal in surgery for nonunions around the elbow is to restore function via secure fixation, assuring union and early mobilization. Disability arises from pain and loss of elbow movement (articular deformity, intra- and extraarticular adhesions, articular cartilage pathology) compounded by instability, weakness, and ulnar nerve neuritis (27).

As disability arises from predictable factors, addressing these will give the best chance of uneventful bony union and a good functional outcome (30). The general approach to treatment consists of the following:

- Restoration of bony stability, alignment, and articular architecture.
- Capsulectomy and ulnar nerve neurolysis.
- Rehabilitation, sometimes including capsular release once union is progressing
- Replacement in the unreconstructable. A desperate attempt to obtain internal fixation of an unrewarding fracture prolongs the operation and exposes the patient to infection and neural injuries.

The anatomy of the distal humerus warrants further consideration. Forming an inverted-Y shape, the medial and laterals columns of the distal humerus make up a triangle with spool-shaped trochlea in between, with the lateral column at 20 degrees and the medial at 40 to 45 degrees to the axis of the humerus. The columns constitute meager skeletal support for the articular surfaces and possess little in the way of soft tissue attachments. The blood supply of the ossification center of the capitellum enters it from the posterior surface, the vessels passing close to the lateral wall of the olecranon fossa (31). These vessels have no communication with the blood supply of the rest of the distal humerus until adulthood. Even then, the basic pattern of the blood supply is maintained, with the addition of intercommunications.

A. Treatment Concepts

There are two possible approaches to the treatment of nonunions around the elbow, in particular with respect to the humeroulnar articulation. One option, and usually the most appropriate, is to restore function via secure fixation. The alternative is total elbow replacement in irreparable trauma. The criteria for fixation are that there be sufficient bone stock to allow stable fixation, that any articular pathology be reversible, and that the patient will be compliant with the rehabilitation program. If these criteria are not met, arthroplasty must be considered. Even in 1980s, range of motion and pain relief were superior in patients who had undergone arthroplasty, but there were problems of loosening in active patients.

B. Clinical Examples

1. Distal Humerus

Nonunion of the Lateral Condyle of the Humerus in Children.   No injury to the lateral humeral condyle in the child can be regarded as trivial. Union is a slower process than in supracondylar fractures; hence adequate immobilization of the fracture must be ensured. Even initially, undisplaced fractures can displace slowly with time, despite cast immobilization, and ultimately fail to unite (32). Debate has existed about the effectiveness of the treatment of nonunion in these fractures, largely based on reports of a high incidence of complication following surgical treatment (33–35). Nonunion is often surprisingly well tolerated by many patients, at least for some time. Surgical correction has in the past been associated with problems of avascular necrosis of the lateral humeral condyle, as well as stiffness. Loss of range of motion remains a problem in the treatment of these nonunions when soft tissue dissection is required. However, by careful choice of approach and, when necessary, staging of the procedure, the risks of avascular necrosis can be reduced.

In the case of delayed union or nonunion less that 12 weeks from the time of injury, there may be little fracture displacement (36). In such circumstances, percutaneous wire or cannulated screw fixation can be used with good results. In Milch type I injuries, as the fracture does not involve the trochlear articulation, long-standing nonunions may result in lateral translation of the lateral humeral condyle rather than angular deformity. Good results can be achieved surgically via a lateral approach sufficient to expose the pseudarthrosis without disturbing the blood supply to the condyle. A peg of bone graft may then be harvested from the proximal ulna and used to supplement the pin fixation of the nonunion (37).

Long-standing nonunion of Milch type II injuries results in a varying amount of lateral rotation and displacement of the lateral humeral condyle, accompanying lateral shift of the ulnar (as the fracture enters the trochlear articulation), worsening valgus deformity, and ulnar nerve neuritis. Lateral angulation can also occur in Milch type I injuries. A staged approach to the treatment of this pattern has been advocated and can be executed with good results (38). First, union of the pseudarthrosis must be achieved, then correction of the angular deformity, and finally ulnar nerve neuritis must be relieved either by transposition, cubital tunnel release, or medial epicondylectomy. Union of the condyle may be achieved in the manner described above. In the case of Milch type I injuries, the angular deformity may be corrected by a simple closing wedge of the medial humerus at the junction of the diaphysis and metaphysis.

A translocation osteotomy is required for the Milch type II injuries in order to avoid unacceptable medial prominence and restore proper alignment of the axes of the humerus and forearm. Both osteotomies can be performed via a posterior approach to the distal humerus, which may also be used to expose the nonunion site. Stabilization of the osteotomy can be difficult, but it can usually be effected with K wires.

In a review of patients 18 years or more after injury, Ippolito reported the results of fractures of the lateral humeral condyle (acute and old) treated depending on the pattern of displacement (39). If tilted, open reduction and K wiring was performed. Among 16 cases, there were 3 poor results: 2 were associated with the development of avascular necrosis and 1 with a varus malunion. Lateral displacement without tilting had been treated without reduction. There were 4 poor results among 20 cases. All of the poor results were seen in displacements of 9 to 10 mm and were associated with 3 nonunions and 1 varus malunion. The 13 cases of old fractures had 10 poor results. Importantly, the results of all excisions of the lateral humeral condyle were poor.

V. NONUNION OF DISTAL HUMERAL FRACTURES IN ADULTS: OPERATIVE TECHNIQUE FOR OPEN REDUCTION AND INTERNAL FIXATION

The last 20 years have shown that great improvements in outcome are possible in the treatment of nonunion in fractures of the distal humerus. Early attempts at dealing with nonunions using K wires and cancellous screws proved to be fraught with problems. Prolonged immobilization was required, and although union was usually achieved, there was little improvement in range of motion. Further procedures were required in 25% of the patients (28). Better results have been achieved by authors successively dealing with the problems of mechanical instability, inadequate articular reduction, and the associated soft tissue problems of peri- and intraarticular fibrosis and ulnar nerve neuritis (30,32,40). In these circumstances, plating of the medial and lateral columns of the distal humerus affords the best chance of achieving stable bone fixation. Adequate exposure of the nonunion is essential and almost always mandates the use of an olecranon osteotomy. Adequate preoperative assessment of ulnar nerve symptoms and signs will determine the need for an ulnar nerve decompression. McGowen's classification (41) is a useful clinical tool to assess and document the severity of the nerve lesion. Grade I is a symptomatic neuritis with no demonstrable motor weakness in the hand, grade III has paralysis of one or more of the ulnar intrinsic hand muscles, and grade II comprises intermediate lesions with weakness but not paralysis.

The standard posterior approach and olecranon osteotomy is used for intercondylar fractures. If only the lateral column is involved, a lateral extensile approach may be utilized. The patient is positioned in the lateral decubitus position with the affected arm up and a tourniquet applied. Whenever possible, old skin incisions are incorporated in to the wound. Olecranon osteotomy is performed in a chevron fashion, taking care to preserve to medial and lateral collateral ligament attachments to the ulna.

The ulnar nerve must be identified in fibrous tissue and adequately mobilized throughout its whole length in the operative field. In the case of ulnar nerve neuritis, a thorough neurolysis can bring about dramatic improvements, both in subjective and objective measurements of outcome (32). The nerve may have to be identified proximally, deep to the triceps, well away from the area of previous surgery. This would usually entail starting the dissection 6 to 8 cm proximal to the medial epicondyle. The use of a loupe or a microscope has been recommended. The distal half of the intermuscular septum is excised, along with encasing fibrous tissue, heterotopic ossification, and any impinging fracture fragments or metalwork. Careful dissection, sparing any motor branches, should be continued for 5 to 6 cm into the pronator muscle group. This strategy has yielded good results, with great patient satisfaction. Even in stage II and III lesions, striking improvements have been reported. No patients were left with residual paralysis and 13 improved from grade II to having no detectable weakness.

Soft tissue fibrosis can then be addressed by resecting posterior periarticular adhesions, together with the fibrotic posterior capsule. If the nonunion is intraarticular, this may then be mobilized to allow access to the anterior capsule for release or resection. Otherwise, dissection can be continued around the lateral aspect of the distal humerus, preserving the lateral ligament complex. Once adequate exposure is achieved, synovectomy is performed, allowing precise definition of the intraarticular nonunion. Malunions may then be osteotomized thru the original fracture lines, and only then can reduction of the fracture fragments be achieved. Temporary K wiring is placed and then definitive plate fixation is performed. Malleable plates are often required due to change in shape of the distal humerus. In the case of bicolumnar fractures, separate lateral and medial column plates should be used, positioned as close to 90 degrees to each other as possible. After a stability test, the olecranon osteotomy is repaired with K wires and a figure-of-eight tension-band wire. The tourniquet should be deflated and hemostasis achieved prior to closing. A well padded posterior splint is applied for 24 hr. Postoperative rehabilitation commences on day 1, with passive flexion and gravity-assisted extension exercises. Active extension can then be commenced at 3 weeks.

In the series of patients reported, the range of motion improved from an arc of 54 degrees to 97 degrees, a great improvement on the result reported for the operative treatment of distal humeral nonunions in the early 1980s. At a mean follow-up of 24 months, there was no progression of degenerative change and ulnar nerve function had consistently improved.

A.   Coonrad-Morrey Semiconstrained Total Elbow Replacement: Operative Technique

Arthroplasty of the elbow represents a solution to the nonunion of the distal humeral fracture in a select group of patients (42). In the elderly, previous unsuccessful treatment may well have led to disuse osteopenia, complicating the preexisting osteoporosis that contributed to the original injury. Often the fracture fragments may be comminuted and very distal. In such circumstances, revision of previously attempted internal fixation is unlikely to yield satisfactory results, even if eventual union is achieved (Fig. 9). The elbow tolerates long periods of immobilization poorly, and this is especially true in the elderly. In the elderly, low-demand patient, excellent pain relief and restoration of function can be achieved by total elbow arthroplasty.

The Coonrad-Morrey total elbow replacement is a semiconstrained sloppy hinge, allowing 7 to 10 degrees of varus/valgus laxity. The stems of the humeral and ulnar components are designed for cemented implantation. The humeral stem also features an anterior flange designed to afford extraosseous cortical fixation, which helps to prevent posterior displacement and resists rotational stresses. The articulation consists of ultrahigh-molecular-weight polyethylene with a linking metal pin.

The procedure is carried out with the patient supine, a tourniquet applied to the limb, and the arm flexed over the chest. Old scars are utilized in the approach, which would otherwise ideally be via a midline posterior approach. The ulnar nerve is identified at the triceps and mobilized sufficiently for its protection. In this approach, the extensor mechanism is left intact, thus facilitating the patient's rehabilitation. The exposure is deepened and the common flexor origin plus the medial collateral ligament are elevated from the medial epicondyle. With elevation of the triceps from the distal humerus, removal of all medial

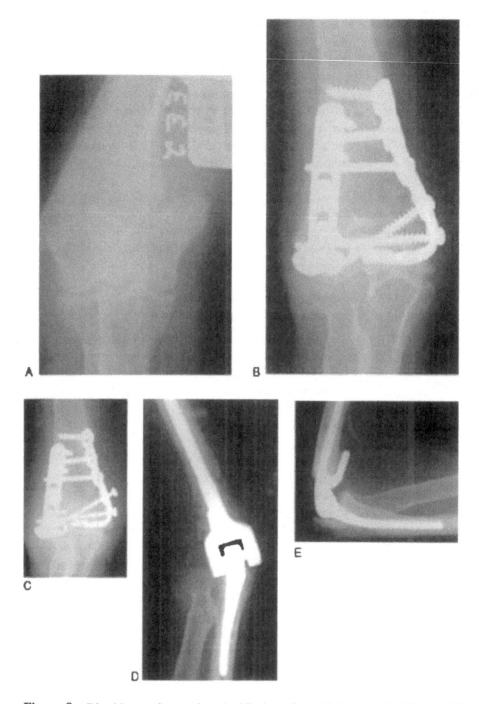

Figure 9   Distal humeral nonunion. A. AP view after initial injury. B. AP view follow-ing open reduction and internal fixation. C. Progressive hardware failure without healing at 3 months. D to F. Total elbow arthoplasty salvage with acceptable functional outcome. (Courtesy of Bruce Ziran, M.D., University of Pittsburgh Medical Center, Pittsburgh, Pennsylvania.)

hardware can be accomplished, along with excision of the fracture fragments. The distal humerus can then be delivered into the exposure, the triceps elevated from the lateral humerus, and the lateral collateral ligament reflected from the bone. Remaining metalwork and fracture fragments can then be removed and the humerus prepared for implantation. The ulnar notch can then be visualized by rotating the forearm. The canal is then prepared. Implantation of the ulnar component is performed first, followed by the humerus, and the two are articulated after the cement has gone off. Rehabilitation can commence as soon as postoperative discomfort allows.

In a review of 36 patients undergoing this procedure for nonunion, significant improvement in performance indices were obtained after surgery. Pain relief was dramatically improved from a starting point where 29 of 36 were in severe pain preoperatively to 31 of 36 with no pain or mild pain postoperatively. The range of motion improved, with the arc of motion progressing from 74 to 111 degrees postoperatively. Deep infection occurred in two cases, one of which was salvaged, the other requiring excision. There were five further complications, including two cases of particulate synovitis, two of ulnar nerve neuritis and one involving a worn bushing. In this specific group of patients, total elbow replacement offers a reliable approach to the relief of pain and restoration of function in nonunion of the distal humerus.

B. Supracondylar Nonunions: Operative Technique

Antegrade humeral nailing has been applied to supracondylar nonunions just above olecranon fossa. In the series presented by Paramasivan (43), 8 patients underwent surgery for painful nonunions in this region. Three patients had one previous attempt at osteosynthesis, three had undergone two previous attempts, and two had had three previous attempts at DCP plate fixation. Olecranon osteotomy was performed and all previous metalwork was removed. Following arthrolysis of the joint, the center of the trochlea was identified and drilled with a 3.2-mm drill, which was then passed proximally across the olecranon fossa and into the intramedullary canal. An antegrade guidewire was then passed in the standard manner, but down to the trochlea. The humerus was then reamed with flexible reamers across the nonunion site and down to the trochlea under direct vision. A humeral nail was the inserted, with the last 8-mm of nail trimmed off to allow very distal locking with long screws. Indeed, 4.5-mm cortical screws were used, as the manufacturer's locking screws were too short. Striking improvement in range of motion was achieved in most patients despite the fact that the nail traversing the olecranon fossa. Three patients underwent subsequent bone grafting; one of these grafts failed to unite. The approach described may be most applicable to the patient who has had several previous procedures, is not infected, and has no intraarticular component. The authors felt that the particular advantage of this approach was to avoid avascular necrosis as a complication of this "bone sandwich."

C. Fine Wire External Fixation: Operative Technique

Infected or contaminated distal humeral fractures represent a particularly difficult management problem. The use of fine-wire external fixation in a previously infected operative field has been shown to give acceptable results from an extremely difficult starting point. Ring (44) describes five cases treated in this way. Four were open fractures in adults treated initially with debridement and fixation, ranging from limited internal fixation with K wires and external fixation to full bicolumnar plating. Initial treatment had to be abandoned in each case because of the development of deep infection. One case was that of a 15-year-old male who had had nonunion of a lateral condylar fracture since the age of 2, which was complicated by an osteotomy with subsequent deep infection. The same operative strategy was used in each case. An olecranon osteotomy was performed via a midline posterior approach, including old scars wherever possible. After ulnar nerve transposition, a tongue and groove was fashioned in the nonunion. The frame construct was of two five-eighth rings posteriorly, connected with four rods. Two distal olive wires were passed at approximately 30 degrees to each other, providing compression at the intercondylar fracture site. Supplementary internal fixation was required in three cases, and two required capsulectomies. The final range of motion was 20 to 130 degrees. Despite the need for further supplementary fixation, the authors felt that this these procedures were performed at a time when a much greater margin of safety was present.

VI. NONUNIONS OF THE RADIAL HEAD AND NECK

Nonunion of fractures to the radial head and neck are uncommon (45). Early excision of comminuted fragments of radial head fractures may well prevent problematic nonunions with loose intraarticular fragments. Nonunion of radial neck fractures, however, is a rare problem but can often be treated conservatively. In the largest reported series of these injuries, Cobb described 6 radial neck fracture nonunions in undisplaced fractures in 5 patients (46). After a period of several months, all regained an excellent range of motion and were essentially asymptomatic. One patient did go on to union after the application of "external bone stimulation." Excision or bone grafting were not recommended as a matter of routine. An expectant policy should be employed and symptomatic problems addressed at a later date, should they arise.

VII. OLECRANON FRACTURES AND OSTEOTOMIES

Nonunion of olecranon fractures was found to occur in up to 5% of cases in the 1970s (47) but had fallen in incidence to approximately 1% in the Mayo Clinic series. Common findings with nonunion of the ulna include decreased range of movement, ulnar neuropathy, posttraumatic OA, and instability. Successful management depends upon achieving fixation, which converts tensile forces around the olecranon (from triceps action) into compressive forces.

Key concepts are as follows:

- To establish whether infection is present
- To determine whether the sigmoid notch is salvageable

Although it was derived from observations made of acute fractures, the Mayo classification is helpful in planning the treatment of established olecranon nonunion. Three variables are considered: displacement, stability, and comminution.

Type I—undisplaced	A. No comminution	B. Minimal comminution
Type II—displaced	A. No comminution	B. Minimal comminution
Type III—unstable	A. No comminution	B. Comminution

In a review of 24 patients with olecranon nonunion, low-energy falls were three times more common as the original injury than was high-energy trauma (48). The principal indication for intervention was pain, and the average movement arc was limited to 86 degrees. Excision of the nonunion fragment was performed only if it involved less than 50% of the olecranon. Surgical fixation was a combined approach of using a DCP plate on the medial aspect and a "bone plate" on the lateral aspect. Union was achieved in 15 of 16 cases treated in this way. None had persisting pain and the average arc of motion improved to 98 degrees (Fig. 10).

In the presence of degenerative changes, nonunion of the olecranon represents a particular challenge. Previously, this had been felt to be a relative contraindication to the use of total elbow replacement (TER) as an alternative to joint reconstruction. However, Papgelopoulos (49) and Gallay (50) have both described the successful use of elbow arthroplasty in these cases. A small fragment can be excised with safety. Larger fragments can be reattached using K wires and tension-band wires or, alternatively, nonabsorbable sutures. Gallay describes leaving a stiff fibrous union intact and performing the arthroplasty through medial and lateral intervals in the triceps. Better visualization is obtained if the nonunion is opened as if it were an osteotomy; the ulnar component is then cemented slightly proud. The olecranon fragment is recessed to accommodate the component. It is then reattached using K wires and tension-band wire, supplemented with an interposition bone graft harvested from the resected radial head when necessary.

Olecranon osteotomy is an essential part of gaining exposure to the intraarticular distal humerus. Transverse osteotomy has been shown to pose a significantly greater risk of nonunion than chevron osteotomy (30 vs. 1%) (51), a finding that has led authors who had reported transverse osteotomies to abandon them in favor of the chevron.

A. Conclusions

Nonunions about the elbow represent a particularly challenging clinical problem. As surgical techniques continue to develop and effective primary treatment be-

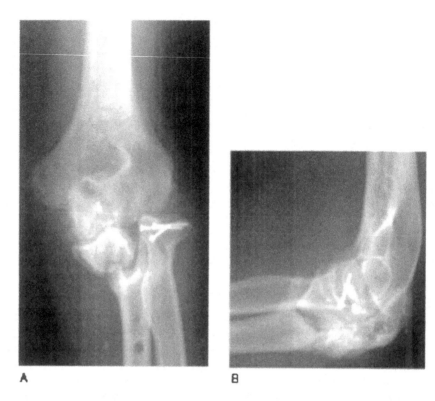

A   B

Figure 10   Infected olecranon nonunion. A and B. Preoperative views after removal of tension-band construct, debridement of infection. (Courtesy of Steven J. Morgan, M.D., Denver Health Medical Center, Denver, Colorado.)

comes more reliable, it is hoped that nonunions will be seen less and less frequently and that useful functional recovery can be achieved more often in those requiring nonunion surgery. Such treatment must address the issues of bony viability and stability hand in hand with measures to release periarticular fibrosis and relieve associated neuritis.

VIII.   NONUNION OF THE FOREARM

During the past 50 years, the incidence of forearm nonunion has dropped dramatically from 46% (52) to 2 to 3% (53,54). In 1949, Knight and Purvis reported a nonunion rate of 46% with open reduction techniques and 12% with closed reduction. Intramedullary Rush nails, which became available in 1957, reduced the nonunion rate to 14% (55). In 1959, Sage developed prebent nails and reported nonunion in only 6% of his patients (56). In 1960, Jinkins (57) published his work using the Eggers plate and reported a nonunion rate of 4%.

Plating of forearm fractures has been described for many decades. Initially, the use of four-holed plates gave disastrous results, with nonunion rates of 40%

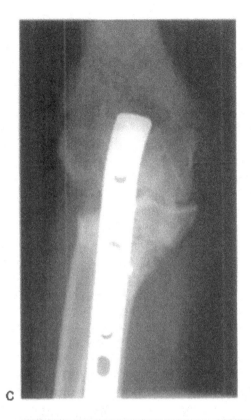

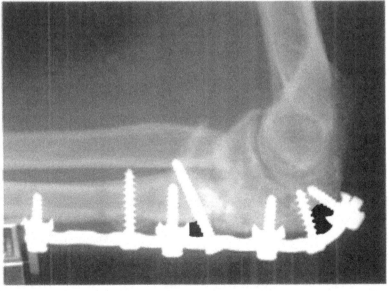

Figure 10 Continued. C and D. Postoperative view of open reduction and internal fixation using Schueli screws to gain purchase and avoid soft tissue stripping. (Courtesy of Steven J. Morgan, M.D., Denver Health Medical Center, Denver, Colorado.)

Table 1 Historical Account of Nonunion Fixation Modalities and Results

Authors	Date	Technique	Failure (%)
Dickson	1944	Kirchner wires	17%
Knight and Purvis	1949	Open reduction	46%
Knight and Purvis	1949	Closed reduction	12%
Evans	1951	Dynamic compression plate	0%
Smith and Sage	1957	IM Nails	14%
Smith and Sage	1957	K wires/Steinmanns pin	38%
Sage	1959	Prebent nails	6%
Jinkins	1960	Eggers plate	4%
Burwell	1964	Dynamic compression plate	0%
Cotler	1971	Schneider nail	6.4%
Weiland	1979	Free fibula	0%
Anderson	1984	Dynamic compression plate	1.4%
Jupiter	1991	Distraction ORIF	0%
Catagni	1994	Ilizarov	0%

(58). The concept of rigid osteosynthesis and the advent of dynamic compression plating in 1969 (59) as well as the accepted use of perioperative antibiotics contributed to improved surgical outcomes (60). In 1984, At the University of Alabama, Anderson (54) reported his experience using a dynamic compression plating (DCP) technique with a nonunion rate of 1.4%. In today's orthopedic world, nonunions are caused by infection, inadequate closed or open reduction (61), and technical errors (62), particularly with hardware insufficient to provide stability (63).

A. Anatomy

An understanding of the forearm anatomy is complementary to the successful management of forearm nonunions. The radius is bowed while the ulna is a straight bone. Sage examined 100 radii (56) and demonstrated four curves within the medullary canal. He also demonstrated that the interosseous membrane, whose fibers run downward and medially from the radius to the ulna, interposed the radius and the ulna. The two bones are connected by an oblique cord, which extends from the radial tuberosity of the radius to the tuberosity of the ulna. The direction of these fibers is opposite to that of the interosseous membrane—i.e., downward and laterally from the ulna to the radius. This anatomical relationship allows the radius to rotate around the ulna along the axis of rotation.

The radius and ulna form a joint proximally maintained by the annular ligament and a joint distally formed by the anterior radioulnar ligaments, posterior radioulnar ligaments, and the triangular fibrocartilage complex.

To achieve a satisfactory functional result of a diaphyseal fracture of the radius and/or ulna:

1. The anatomical relationship between the radius and the ulna must be restored.
2. The interosseous membrane is an important factor in maintaining the stability between the radius and ulna; this is the basis for maintaining the interosseous space to achieve a good result.
3. Axial and rotational alignment should be achieved, as this restores pronation and supination.

B. Definition of Nonunion in the Forearm

A forearm fracture is classified as a nonunion when at least 9 months have elapsed and the fracture has not shown progressive signs of healing for 3 months. The time factor can differ according to the type of the fracture; hence this definition is controversial.

There are three main types of nonunions in the forearm: hypertrophic or hyperactive vascular nonunion, oligotrophic nonunion, and atrophic or avascular nonunion. Hypertrophic nonunion is a result of inadequate surgical technique, improper fixation, or premature motion at the fracture site. Oligotrophic nonunions have no callus and occur because of major fracture displacement combined with fragment distraction and internal fixation without proper fragment apposition. Atrophic nonunions result from decreased vascularity from infection, severe soft tissue damage, or overenthusiastic exposure of bone fragments at the time of surgery (60). Compromised blood supply combined with inadequate reduction or fixation is a sure recipe for the development of an atrophic forearm nonunion.

C. Treatment

The prognosis for forearm nonunion before the mid-nineteenth century was not particularly hopeful owing to the nonavailability of radiography and lack of proper fixation techniques and devices (64). Consequently, forearm nonunions were not treated because the recognized forms of treatment involved considerable risk (65). In those early days, multiple treatment strategies were available, including friction between the two ends of bone to stimulate healing (66), resection of the ends of the bones (66), indirect irritation of bones by the application of stimulating agents, and electricity and galvanism. Smith in 1855 used weight-bearing braces (67), while Thomas (68) in the late 1800s suggested that daily percussion with a hammer and damming (venous congestion imposed by venous tourniquet) enhanced healing.

Forearm nonunions need individual analysis of the reason for their occurrence and a different treatment approach must be designed for each case. In acute fractures, a closed reduction with remaining displacement of the fracture fragments will end in nonunion in a high percentage of cases (61). Currently, open reduction and internal fixation of displaced both-bone forearm fractures in the adult is considered standard to avoid nonunion (69).

Once a nonunion has occurred and the underlying cause has been diagnosed, a variety of treatment options are available, including open reduction, internal fixation with bone grafting, intramedullary fixation, external fixation, distraction osteogenesis, and free vascularized bone transfer.

1. Internal Fixation

Sufficient stability without excessive rigidity should be the aim in treating forearm nonunions. It is recommended to have at least six to eight cortices using 3.5-mm dynamic compression plating (70,71). One purpose of the plate is neutralization of torsional forces. Since the radius describes an important excursion around the ulna during rotation, the plate must be long enough to achieve control and reduce the lever arm of torsional force at the fracture site (61). The 3.5-mm plates provide adequate stability without impeding motion of the forearm or causing excessive stress shielding. Low-contact dynamic compression plates reduce the bone/plate interface, allow for compression at the nonunion site, and minimize inhibition of local cortical blood flow.

Oligotrophic nonunions may require a bone graft in addition to plating. Atrophic nonunions absolutely require bone grafting, bone graft substitute, or transfer of a free or vascularized segment of bone—depending upon the gap size—if plating is to be successful. A volar approach to the radius and a subcutaneous ulnar approach provide adequate exposure while minimizing iatrogenic damage to the posterior interosseous nerve. For compression plating to be effective, compression at the nonunion site must be achieved. For each screw placed in compression mode, 1 mm of compression is achieved. If necessary, a tensioning device can be used, with additional surgical exposure as needed. The rigidity of a plate construct is increased tremendously with the addition of interfragmentary or axial bone compression. If compression is not achieved in forearm nonunion surgery, then the goals of surgery have not been met and failure is likely.

IX. NONUNION OF BOTH RADIUS AND ULNA

If it is necessary to achieve congruent surfaces, bone ends can be resected within 2 cm of shortening. Compression plating can then treat the nonunions. Defects in the proximal third of the radius or the distal 5 to 8 cm of the ulna can be treated by excision of the fragments (60). It is simpler to remove the fragments than to graft them.

Unequal lengths of the radius and or ulna can be a threat in treating forearm nonunions and can reduce pronation supination or make the movements painful.

X. RADIAL OR ULNAR NONUNIONS ALONE

Rates of nonunion of isolated ulnar shaft fractures have ranged from 0.08 to 12% (72). The ulna remains the most difficult bone in the body in which to achieve primary healing due to the torsional stresses during pronosupination (71). Compression plating via a direct approach between the flexor carpi ulnaris and extensor carpi ulnaris is recommended. Brackenburg has reported union rates of over 92% using this technique (73). After fractures of radius and ulna, a situation can arise wherein either the radius or the ulna has not healed. Excising the ends of the nonunion and bone grafting with compression plating treats this situation. If one bone has not healed with the other one in malunion, the treatment is simpler: the ends of the malunited bone and the ununited bone are excised to equalize the length of the forearm. Compression plating and bone grafting are used to stabilize the fragments.

XI.   ISOLATED LARGE RADIAL
OR ULNAR DEFECTS

Isolated large radial or ulnar injuries are rare but can be seen after high-velocity injuries such as those due to gunshots or following infection. Twin-onlay cortical fibular struts screwed together, cancellous bone grafts, vascularized fibular grafts, tricortical iliac crest grafts, or bone transport achieves stability (60,74). With massive single bone defects either in the radius or the ulna, a single-bone forearm can be created.

A.   Bone Grafting

Bone grafting is required in most forearm nonunions. Currently the techniques most performed are cancellous autografts, whole fibular grafts (vascularized and nonvascularized), and tricortical strut grafts (75). With defects of less than 2.5 cm, cancellous bone grafting is useful. The use of cancellous bone grafting in nonunions of the tibias is reported to be 92% successful (73). With larger defects, tricortical or whole fibular strut grafts are used. With defects larger than 5 to 6 cm, vascularized fibular grafts have been introduced.

B.   Osseous Transplants

Large-defect nonunions in the radius and ulna can be treated successfully with whole fibular transplants. Vascularized fibular transfer is a valuable technique for reconstructing extensive long bone defects in the upper extremity. A successfully transplanted autogenous fibular graft is a viable bone (Fig. 11). The osteocytes and osteoblasts survive, and because of the preservation of bone-forming capacity, bone fusion occurs early (76). The fibula's tubular shape is similar to the shape of the forearm and does not overstuff the forearm (76–78). In recent years, many reports of skeletal reconstruction using free vascularized fibula for forearm nonunions have been published (79–82). Weiland reported five patients, four of whom had primary bone union (83). Olekas reported a series of 15 patients, 11 (73%) of whom had primary union within 3 to 6 months after the operation (77).

C.   Bone Transport (Ilizarov) and Distraction

Hypotrophic nonunions have been treated successfully with compression using the Ilizarov ring fixator. The concept of distraction osteogenesis, using the Ili-

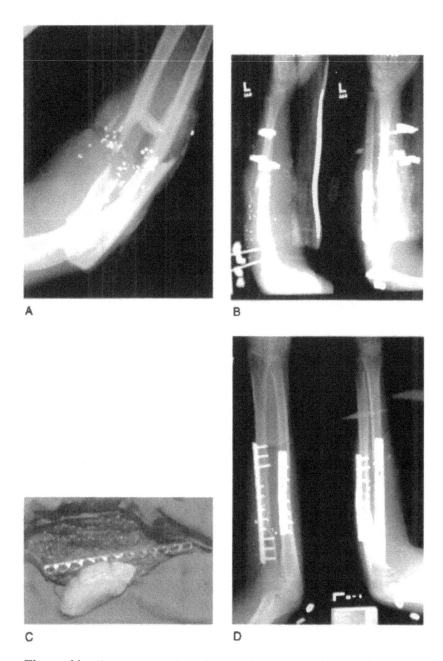

Figure 11 Forearm nonunion after gunshot wound with infection and bone loss. A. Initial x-ray after time of injury. B. X-rays after prolonged external fixation. C. Transfer of vascularized osteocutaneous fibular graft with plate fixation. D. Early healing at 4 months. (Courtesy of Steven Peterson, M.D., Denver Health Medical Center, Denver, Colorado.)

zarov method, also permits simultaneous correction of axial deformity, angular deformity, translational deformity, shortening, bone loss, and infection (84) (Fig. 12).

Limb distraction techniques have been described since 1903 (85). Kravchuk described the concept of distraction through an area of hypertrophic bony union in 1976 (86). Both Ilizarov and Catagni proposed that the stable environment created with the Ilizarov fixation would lead to union in hypertrophic nonunions.

Catagni reported a series of 21 patients with hypertrophic forearm nonunions treated by using the Ilizarov apparatus in distraction; he concluded that distraction osteogenesis offered the most complete method of providing optimal limb function (87).

Jupiter reported a unique method for the treatment of a complex malpositioned nonunion of the radius by means of intraoperative distraction. His surgical

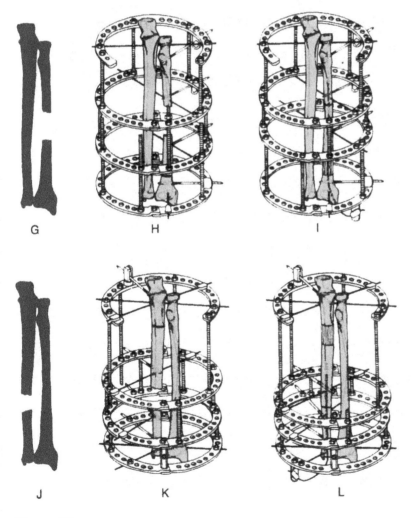

Figure 12

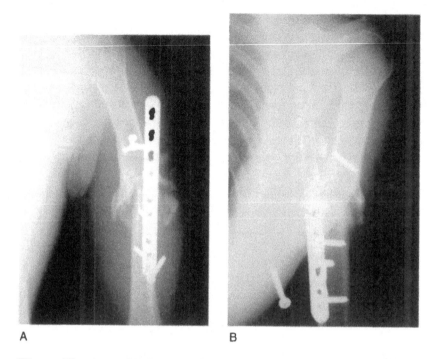

A   B

Figure 13   A and B. Hypertrophic nonunion with hardware failure.

technique combined indirect reduction and intraoperative distraction of the radius by means of a femoral distractor with conventional grafting of autogenous iliac crest bone and AO plating (88). This technique addressed the functional length, alignment, and restoration of the distal radioulnar joint and interosseous space and hence afforded the patients stability and functional forearm rotation.

XII. SUMMARY

Diaphyseal nonunions of the radius and ulna present certain difficulties. The recovery of function after a fracture of both bones of the forearm is dependent on the return of rotation of the forearm and the maintenance of a functional range of motion of the wrist and elbow. Significant functional deficits ensue if these anatomical parameters are not restored.

The goals of surgery in treating forearm nonunions are restoring alignment, radial bow, and length; allowing for early functional rehabilitation; and achieving a stable yet biologically sound construct.

Open reduction and internal fixation is the standard for the majority of forearm nonunions, but there is an important role for other techniques, such as distraction osteogenesis and vascularized fibular transfer in cases with infection or bone loss.

REFERENCES

1. AO Principles of Fracture Management. Stuttgart and New York: Ruedi, Murphy-Thieme, 2000, pp 121–127.
2. A Sarmiento, JB Zagorski, GA Zych, LL Latta, CA Capps. Functional bracing for the treatment of fractures of the humeral diaphysis. J Bone Surg Am 2000 82(4): 478–486.
3. A Barquet, A Fernandez, J Luvozio, R Masliah. A combined therapeutic protocol for aseptic nonunion of the humeral shaft: A report of 25 cases. J Trauma 1989; 29:95–98.
4. HA Fattah, EE Halawa, TH Shafy. Nonunion of the humeral shaft: A report on 25 cases. Injury 1982; 14:225–262.
5. H Rosen. The treatment of nonunions and pseudarthroses of the humeral shaft. Orthop Clin North Am 1990; 21:725–742.
6. R Loomer, P Kokan. Nonunion in fractures of the humeral shaft. Injury 1976; 7: 274–278.
7. MA Catagni, F Guerreschi, RA Probe. Treatment of humeral nonunions with the Ilizarov technique. Bull Hosp Jt Dis Orthop Inst 1991; 51:74–83.
8. NO Christensen. Kuntcher intramedullary reaming and nail fixation for nonunion of the humerus. Clin Orthop 1976; 116:225–5.
9. JB Jupiter. Complex non-union of the humeral dyaphysis. J Bone Joint Surg (Am) 72:701–707, 1990.
10. CC Wu, CH Shih. Treatment for nonunion of the shaft of the humerus: Comparison of plates and Seidel interlocking nails. Can J Surg 1992; 35:661–665.
11. W Healy, GM White, CA Mick, AF Brooker, AJ Weiland. Nonunion of the humeral shaft. Clin Orthop 1987; 219:206–213.
12. CY Chen, SW Ueng, CH Shih. Staged management of infected humeral nonunion. J Trauma 1997;43:793–798.
13. J Lammens, G Bauduin, R Driesen, et al: Treatment of nonunion of the humerus using the Ilizarov external fixator. Clin Orthop 1998; 353:223–230.
14. J Lin, SM Hou, YS Hang. Locked nailing for humeral shaft delayed unions and nonunions. J Trauma 2000;48:695–703.
15. S Hoppenfeld, P De Boer. Surgical Exposure in Orthopaedics, 2nd ed., Philadelphia: Lippincott, 1994, pp 51–82.
16. WJ Mills, DP Hanel, DG Smith. Lateral approach to the humeral shaft: An alternative approach for fracture treatment. J Orthop Trauma 1996; 10(2):81–86.
17. TR Guse, RF Ostrum. The surgical anatomy of the radial nerve around the humerus. Clin Orthop 1995; 320:149–153.
18. AF Farragos, EH Schemitsch, MD McKee. Complications of intramedullary nailing for fractures of the humeral shaft: a review. J Orthop Trauma 1999; 13:258–267.
19. J Lin, SM Hou. Antegrade locked nailing for humeral shaft fractures. Clin Orthop 1999; 365:201–210.
20. G Pietu, G Raynaud, J Letenneur. Treatment of delayed and nonunions of the humeral shaft using the Seidel locking nail: A preliminary report of five cases. J Orthop Trauma 1994; 8:240–244.
21. M Raschke, C Khodadadyan, PD Maitino, R Hoffmann, NP Sudkamp. Nonunion of the humerus following intramedullary nailing treated by Ilizarov hybrid fixation. J Orthop Trauma 1998; 12:138–141.

22. T Flinkkila, J Ristiniemi, M Hamalainen. Nonunion after intramedullary nailing of humeral shaft fractures. J Trauma 2001; 50:540–544.

23. MD McKee, MA Miranda, BL Riemer, et al. Management of humeral nonunion after the failure of locking intramedullary nails. J Orthop Trauma 1996;10:492–499.

24. J Lin, N Inoue, A Valdevit, et al. Biomechanical comparison of antegrade and retrograde nailing of humeral shaft fractures. Clin Orthop 1998; 351:203–213.

25. R Cattaneo, MA Catagni, F Guerreschi. Applications of the Ilizarov method in the humerus: Lengthenings and nonunions. Hand Clin 1993;9:729–739.

26. C Cuiccarelli, C Cervellati, G Montanari, et al. The Ilizarov method for the treatment of nonunion in the humerus. Chir Organi Mov 1990; 75:115–120. JL Esterhai.

27. VR, OK Menan, RD Pool, RB Simons. Nonunion of the humerus after failure & surgical treatment, Management using the Ilizarov circular tractor. J Bone Joint Surg Br 2000; 82(7):977–983.

28. J Sodergard, J Sandelin, O Bostman. Postoperative complications of distal humeral fractures. 27/96 adults followed up for 6 (2–10) years. Acta Orthop Scand 1992; 63(1):85–89.

29. MM Mitsunaga, RS Bryan, RL Linscheid. Condylar nonunions of the elbow. J Trauma 1982; 22(9):787–791.

30. M McKee, J Jupiter, CL Toh, L Wilson, C Colton, KK Karras. Reconstruction after malunion and nonunion of intra-articular fractures of the distal humerus. Methods and results in 13 adults. J Bone Joint Surg Br 1994; 76(4):614–621.

31. JB Jupiter. Complex fractures of the distal part of the humerus and associated complications. Instr Course Lect 1995; 44:187–198.

32. S Haraldsson. The intraosseous vasculature of the distal end of the humerus with special reference to the capitellum. Acta Orthop Scand 1957; 27:81–93.

33. JC Flynn, JF Richards Jr, RI Saltzman. Prevention and treatment of non-union of slightly displaced fractures of the lateral humeral condyle in children. An end-result study. J Bone Joint Surg Am 1975; 57(8):1087–1092.

34. JS Speed, HB Macey. Fracture of the humeral condyles in children. J Bone Joint Surg 1933, 15:569–572.

35. KS Dhillon, S Sengupta, BJ Singh. Delayed management of fracture of the lateral humeral condyle in children. Acta Orthop Scand 1988; 59(4):419–424.

36. JA Hardacre, SH Nahigian, AI Froimson, JR Brown. Fractures of the lateral condyle of the humerus in children. J Bone Joint Surg Am 1971; 53(6):1083–1089.

37. R Papandrea, PM Waters. Posttraumatic reconstruction of the elbow in the pediatric patient. Clin Orthop 2000; 370:115–126.

38. JC Flynn. Nonunion of slightly displaced fractures of the lateral humeral condyle in children: an update. J Pediatr Orthop 1989; 9(6):691–696.

39. KE Wilkins. Residuals of elbow trauma in children. Orthop Clin North Am 1990; 21(2):291–314.

40. E Ippolito, C Tudisco, P Farsetti, R Caterini. Fracture of the humeral condyles in children: 49 cases evaluated after 18–45 years. Acta Orthop Scand 1996; 67(2): 173–178.

41. G Ackerman, JB Jupiter. Non-union of fractures of the distal end of the humerus. J Bone Joint Surg Am 1988; 70(1):75–83.

42. AJ McGowen. The results of transposition of the ulna nerve for traumatic ulnar neuritis: J Bone Joint Surg Br 1950; 32:293–301.

43. MD McKee, JB Jupiter, G Bosse, L Goodman. Outcome of ulnar neurolysis during post-traumatic reconstruction of the elbow. J Bone Joint Surg Br 1998; 80(1):100–105.

44. BF Morrey, RS Adams. Semiconstrained elbow replacement for distal humeral nonunion. J Bone Joint Surg Br 1995; 77(1):67–72.

45. ON Paramasivan, DA Younge, R Pant. Treatment of nonunion around the olecranon fossa of the humerus by intramedullary locked nailing. J Bone Joint Surg Br 2000; 82(3):332–335.

46. D Ring, JB Jupiter, S Toh. Salvage of contaminated of the distal humerus with thin wire external fixation. Clin Orthop 1999; (359):203–208.

47. G Horne, P Sim. Nonunion of the radial head. J Trauma 1985; 25(5):452–453.

48. TK Cobb, RD Beckenbaugh. Nonunion of the radial neck following fracture of the radial head and neck: Case reports and a review of the literature. Orthopedics 1998; 21(3):364–368.

49. PJ Mayer, CM Evarts. Nonunion, delayed union, malunion and avascular necrosis. In: CH Epps Jr, ed. Complications in Orthopaedic surgery. Vol. 1. Philadelphia: Lippincott, 1978, pp 159–175.

50. PJ Papagelopoulos, BF Morrey. Treatment of nonunion of olecranon fractures. J Bone Joint Surg Br 1994; 76(4):627–635.

51. SH Gallay, MD McKee. Operative treatment of nonunions about the elbow. Clin Orthop 2000; (370):87–101.

52. BJ Gainor, F Moussa, T Schott. Healing rate of transverse osteotomies of the olecranon used in reconstruction of distal humerus fractures. J South Orthop Assoc 1995; 4(4):263–268.

53. RA Knight, GD Purvis. Fractures of both bones of the forearm in adults. J Bone Joint Surg [A] 1949; 31A: 755–764.

54. LD Anderson, DW Bacastow. Treatment of forearm shaft fractures with compression plates. Contemp Orthop 1984; 8:17–25.

55. LD Anderson, TD Sisk, RE Tooms, WI Park III. Compresion-plate fixation in acute diaphyseal fractures of the radius and ulna. J Bone Joint Surg [A] 1975; 57-A: 287–297.

56. H Smith, FP Sage. Medullary fixation of forearm fractures. J Bone Joint Surg [A] 1957; 39-A: 91–98.

57. FP Sage. Medullary fixation of fractures of the forearm: A study of the medullary canal of the radius and a report of fifty fractures of the radius treated with a prebent triangular nail. J Bone Joint Surg [A] 1959; 41-A: 1489–1516.

58. WJ Jinkins Jr, LD Leckhart, GWN Eggers. Fractures of the forearm in adults. South Med J 1960; 53: 669–679.

59. JG Caden. Internal fixation of fractures of the forearm. J Bone Joint Surg [A] 1961; 43-A: 1115–1121.

60. SM Perren, M Russenberger, S Steinmann, et al. A dynamic compression plate. Acta Orthop Scand Suppl 1969; 125: 31–41.

61. G Gruen, MA Pappas. Malunion and nonunion. In: J Herndon, ed. Surgical Reconstruction of the Upper Extremity. Stamford, CT: Appleton & Lange, 19XX, pp 349–359.

62. RB Heppenstall, CT Brighton, JL Esterhai Jr, et al. Clinical and roentgenographic evaluation of non-union of the forearm in relation to treatment with DC electrical stimulation. J Trauma 1983; 23(8):740–744.
63. U Heim, R Zehnder. Analyse von misserfolgen nach Osteosynthesen von Unterarm-schaftfracturen. Hefte Unfallheilkd 1989; 210:243–258.
64. JA Rosacker, JA Kopta. Both bone fractures of the forearm: A review of surgical variables associated with union. Orthopedics 1981; 4:1353.
65. RA Brandt, CT Rubin. Fracture healing. In: C McCollister, ed. Surgery of the Musculoskeletal System. New York: Churchill Livingstone, 1997, pp 93–114.
66. J Syme. The Principles of Surgery. Edinburgh: Maclachan and Stewart, 1832.
67. EM Bick. Source Book of Orthopaedics. New York: Hafner, 1968.
68. H Smith. On the treatment of ununited dracture by means of artificial limbs, which combine the principle of pressure and motion at the seat of the fracture, and lead to the formation of the unsheathing callus. Am J Med Sci 1855; 29:102.
69. HO Thomas. Contribution to Surgery and Medicine. The Principles of Treatment of Fractures and Dislocations. Part VI. London: HK Lewis, 1886.
70. D Bell, JN Keelam. Nonunions and malunions of the upper extremity. In: Chapman MW. ed. Operative Orthopaedics. Philadelphia: Lippincott, 1988, pp 529–543.
71. ME Muller, M Allgower, R Schneider, H Willeneger. Manual of Forearm Fixation. Berlin: Springer-Verlag, 1979.
72. PJ Stern, WJ Drury. Complications of plate fixation of forearm fractures. Clin Orthop 1983;175:25–29.
73. F Pollock, AM Parkovich, JJ Prieto, et al. The islolated fracture of the ulnar shaft. J Bone Joint Surg [A] 1983; 65-A: 339.
74. PH Brakenburg, JR Corea, ME Blackmore. Non-union of the isolated fracture of the ulnar shaft in adults. Injury 1981; 12:371.
75. RD Esser. Treatment of a bone defect of the forearm by bone transport. Clin Orthop Rel Res 1996;326:221–224.
76. PC Dell, JE Shepphard. Vascularized bone grafts in the treatment of infected fore-arm nonunions. J Hand Surg [A] 1984; 9(5):653–658.
77. T Hirayama, N Suematsu, et al. Free vascularised bone graft in reconstruction of the upper extremity. J Hand Surg [Br] 1985; 10(2):169–175.
78. J Olekas, A Guobys. Vascularised bone transfer for defect and pseudarthroses of forearm bones. J Hand Surg [Br] 1991; 16(4):406–408.
79. MB Wood. Upper extremity reconstruction by vascularized bone transfers: Results and complications. J Hand Surg [A] 1987; 12(3):422–427.
80. RWH Pho. Free vascularized fibular transplant for replacement of the lower radius. J Bone Joint Surg [Br] 1979; 61:362–365.
81. Y Allieu, R Gomis, et al. Congenital pseudarthrosis of the forearm—Two cases treated by vascularized fibular graft. J Hand Surg [A]1981; 6:475–481.
82. LC Hurst, MA Mirza, et al. Vascularised fibular graft for infected loss of the ulna. Case report. J Hand Surg [A] 1982; 7:498–501.
83. PC Dell, JE Sheppard. Vascularised bone grafts in the treatment of infected forearm nonunions. J Hand Surg [A] 1984; 9:653–658.
84. AJ Weiland, HE Kleinert, JE Kutz, RK Daniel. Free vascularized bone grafts in surgery of the upper extremity. J Hand Surg [A] 1979; 34:129–144.
85. R Aldegheri, G Tessari. Disugualianza radio-ulnar. Minerva Ortop 1985; 6:707.

86.   VL Kravchuk. Clinico-reontgenographic dynamics of the reparative regeneration in conditions of distraction in pseudarthroses of tubular bones of the lower extremities (trans). Orthop Travmatol Protez 1976; 36:28.
87.   MA Catagni, F Guerreschi, JA Holman, R Cattaneo. Distraction osteogenesis in the treatment of stiff hypertrophic nonunions using the Ilizarov apparatus. Clin Orthop 1994; 301:159–163.
88.   JB Jupiter, T Ruedi. Intraoperative distraction in the treatment of complex nonunions of the radius. J Hand Surg [A] 1992; 17–3:416–422.

7

Polytrauma and Open Fracture of the Upper Extremity

**Greg M. Osgood, Vishal Sarwahi,
and Melvin P. Rosenwasser**
*New York Orthopaedic Hospital, Columbia-Presbyterian Medical Center,
New York, New York, U.S.A.*

I. INTRODUCTION

Care of patients with traumatic injuries has evolved dramatically within the past decade. The tenets of trauma management, however, remain virtually unchanged. Reevaluation of trauma protocols has yielded standardized methods of treating patients with multiple injuries. The severity of injury and complexity of poly-trauma demands a systematic approach to treatment. Applying the principles of orthopedic polytrauma to patients with severe open injuries allows the surgeon to predict outcomes.

Level 1 trauma centers currently face an increasing number of open upper extremity injuries from two sources: blunt trauma associated with motor vehicle accidents (MVAs) and penetrating ballistic injuries. Both types of injury are commonly associated with complex disruptions of the soft tissue envelope involving compromised nerves, vascular supply, and musculotendinous units. Blunt MVA trauma often involves multiple system injury and multiple affected extremities.

II. OPEN FRACTURES OF THE UPPER EXTREMITY RESULT FROM HIGH-ENERGY INJURY

A. Motor Vehicle Trauma

The evolution of motor vehicles has mirrored the increasing public attention to safety. New technologies in automotive design, safety testing, passenger protection, and road design have significantly decreased the incidence of fatal MVAs. Improvements in automotive safety devices—including seat design modifications, the combined lap and shoulder restraint, and the air bag—have decreased the number of life-threatening accidents. The use of seat belts and air bags has decreased death by 86%, the likelihood of severe injury (injury severity score >15) by 61%, and the incidence of major surgery or the need for surgery by 48% (1). Improved engine and safety engineering, crumple zones, and insulation materials have further improved car safety.

Road safety studies have prompted changes in road layout. The conversion of intersections from signals to roundabouts can lead to a 76% decrease in injury-causing accidents and a 90% decrease in MVA fatalities at these locations (2). Flail chests, pulmonary and cardiac contusions, intraabdominal vascular injuries, quadriplegic events, and fatalities are much less common results of MVAs. Crashes that would otherwise have caused numerous deaths now result in polytrauma and limb-threatening injuries. Patients present to the emergency room unstable but alive. The fallout from this is a decrease in the number of patients dead on arrival and a relative increase in the number of surviving complex trauma and polytrauma patients arriving at major trauma centers worldwide. Additionally, advances in orthopedic surgery have made the treatment of certain injuries a priority and a possibility in the acute setting; delaying operative management has been found to offer no significant benefit.

B. Penetrating Ballistic Injuries

Injuries caused by firearm missiles are classified as due to either low- or high-velocity missiles based on the missile's exit speed: low-velocity rounds generally have a speed of 1000 ft/s, whereas a high-velocity round is defined as one with a speed of 2000 ft/s or above. The trauma caused is proportional to the kinetic energy of the missile and therefore proportional to the square of the velocity. Most handguns are considered low-velocity weapons. Low-energy ballistics inflict a smaller zone of injury, often limited to moderate soft tissue damage and minimally comminuted fractures. High-velocity missiles, however, inflict devastating, widespread destruction of the soft tissues, complex comminuted fractures, and organ damage. These injuries extend to distant areas of the body through an inconstant vector. The increasing availability of legal and illegal firearms increases the likelihood of high-velocity ballistic injuries presenting to trauma centers. These weapons are often the source of upper extremity open fracture and complex trauma. Combat injuries are often caused by explosives and shrapnel, which may be considered high-velocity weapons; they are associated with higher degrees of soft tissue injury from thermal burns, the high energy of the explosive blast, and the number of penetrating particles (3).

III. EVALUATION OF THE POLYTRAUMA PATIENT

Upper extremity trauma may occur as an isolated injury or as part of a constellation of injuries in the context of polytrauma. The polytrauma patient is managed in a systematic manner, which is part of a universal management protocol at trauma centers. Standardization of care in the field and in the hospital has improved communication and flow of care in the setting of acute trauma.

Treatment of the polytrauma patient can be approached as five phases of care: resuscitation, emergency procedures, stabilization, delayed operative procedures, and rehabilitation (4).

A. Phases of Trauma Care

1. Resuscitation

The evaluation and management of patients in the resuscitation phase are guided by the accepted standards of Advanced Trauma Life Support (ATLS) protocols. This phase begins when the patient is first evaluated in the field by emergency medical technicians and paramedics and should be well under way when the patient arrives in the emergency room (ER). It concludes when the patient is hemodynamically stable. A trauma patient's airway competency, ability to breathe, and circulatory stability, known as the ABCs, are assessed and treated. The ABCs remain the cornerstone for prevention of early death following trauma.

The oropharynx must be cleared of debris or injured tissue and the conduit to the lungs must be established and protected. Oropharyngeal and nasopharyngeal airways are used to protect an existing airway. Rarely is a tracheostomy required to establish an airway. Guarding this pathway is especially important in patients who have suffered inhalation injuries and blunt head and neck trauma. These patients may present with an airway and may be breathing on initial examination; however, their airways are in jeopardy due to laryngeal edema. Constant reevaluation is mandatory. The trauma team must be equipped to intubate a patient whose airway becomes compromised. Gentle in-line cervical traction or a jaw-thrust maneuver performed by an assistant may be safely used to open the airway or facilitate intubation in patients who have sustained neck trauma.

Once the airway is cleared, spontaneous or assisted breathing must be established. The assessment of breathing includes an evaluation of the quality of breathing. Labored breathing should be supported while the cause is being determined. This may require sedation and paralysis in the acute setting to optimize oxygenation. If manual ventilation with a bag-valve-mask device is ineffective, an inadequate airway, hemothorax, or pneumothorax is suggested. Correction of a malpositioned endotracheal tube and immediate decompression of the chest cavity will resolve these conditions. In the prehospital setting, needle thoracostomy above the second rib in the line of the nipple releases pressure in the affected hemithorax. In the emergency room, this is replaced with tube thoracostomy in the axillary line.

The circulatory assessment begins with measurement of vital signs. Hypovolemia—manifest as hypotension and tachycardia—is treated with the rapid infusion of intravenous fluids. Two large-bore intravenous lines are inserted. A single bolus of 1000 mL of lactated Ringer's solution is administered and repeated if vital signs do not correct. Serial hematocrits determine the severity of ongoing bleeding. Blood should be cross-matched and used when available; however, in the emergent setting of a falling hematocrit and hypotension type O negative blood should be administered to correct persistent hemodynamic instability. The assessment of circulation is not complete until the patient is stabilized or a source of bleeding is found. External sources of bleeding should respond to direct pressure. If no source of external bleeding is identified, deep peritoneal lavage should be performed by the general surgery members of the trauma team. Internal bleeding in the abdominal cavity or the pelvis is further evaluated with angiography and may require embolization to establish patient stability.

Most trauma protocols include a rapid neurological assessment, important in the prevention of early death. The Glasgow Coma Scale is universally used to communicate a patient's level of consciousness, verbal response, and motor control (5). Pupillary response, motor coordination, sensory function, and rectal tone are documented. Serial examinations are important in following the evolution of a patient's injuries. A rapid deterioration in central nervous function requires acute computed tomography (CT) of the head for evaluation and signals a need for neurosurgical intervention.

The resuscitation phase concludes when the patient is hemodynamically stable and shock is treated. This allows further evaluation of injuries that place the patient at risk for continued blood loss.

2. Emergency Procedures

The indication for early emergency surgery in the trauma patient is persistent instability, which cannot be rectified without operative intervention. This includes significant vascular injury, lacerations of the abdominal viscera, depressed fractures of the skull, progressive neurological compromise, and continued hemodynamic instability secondary to pelvic fracture. The application of a pelvic external fixator decreases pelvic bleeding and stabilizes the patient during transportation. Femoral fractures and significant pelvic injuries should be repaired early to prevent pulmonary decompensation. Femoral fractures are treated with external fixation or intramedullary rodding. Emergency procedures are also performed in this phase for prophylaxis against pulmonary failure (6–9). Finally, extremity surgery and splinting are required in this phase to diminish the potential for additional neural injury following unstable fractures, including scapulothoracic dissociation, clavicular fractures, fracture/dislocations about the proximal humerus, and humeral shaft fractures.

3. Stabilization

The principles of resuscitation and indications for early surgery are still of paramount importance throughout the stabilization phase. Open fractures are treated emergently once the patient is stable. Long bone fractures and pelvic fractures that have not yet been stabilized are treated during this phase. Operative intervention for open fractures in the stabilization phase is directed toward decreasing the likelihood of hemodynamic instability that may result from fracture. This includes external fixation of long bone fractures of the lower extremity or definitive fixation (depending on the patient's condition) during washout of the soft tissue injury. Most orthopedic injuries, however, must wait until the patient is medically stable and optimized for surgery; these definitive procedures should not be performed during the stabilization phase.

Patient care during the stabilization phase is best performed in the surgical intensive care unit, where ventilation can be mechanically supported, vital signs are measured continuously, and central venous and peripheral arterial lines can be supported. The adequacy of therapy is gauged by stable vital signs, laboratory studies, urine output, and especially the absence of coagulopathy.

4. Delayed Operative Procedures

Once the patient is hemodynamically stable, he or she is returned to the OR for required surgical procedures. Injuries are prioritized and treated in an order that will minimize the risk of additional complications associated with the injury. Open fractures undergo irrigation and debridement every 48 to 72 h. Soft tissue coverage and closure should be performed as early as possible to decrease further soft tissue dehydration and necrosis (especially articular cartilage and neurovascular structures) and to minimize the risk of secondary infection and systemic sepsis.

During the stabilization and delayed operative procedures phases, the trauma team must pay careful attention to the patient's nutritional status. Nutritional consultation is useful in providing adequate calories and nutrients to balance the patient's increased catabolic rate by the best route. Laboratory indicators, such as lymphocyte count and serum albumin, are helpful in assessing progress.

5. Recovery and Rehabilitation

At the conclusion of the operative phase, physical therapy, occupational therapy, and social work play vital roles in minimizing disability. Recovery is often the longest of the five phases; therefore, continued nutritional assessment and psychosocial evaluation are critical in preserving function and patient motivation. Transfer to a rehabilitation center that specializes in individual elements of recuperation is beneficial.

B. Identifying the Injury

The polytrauma patient must be assessed with regard to the overall injury in addition to the severity of individual insults. This helps the traumatologist to select the most appropriate treatment for different elements of polytrauma in an effort to optimize the patient's overall function at the end of rehabilitation. In this light, the global injury and each component are assessed by standard methods.

1. Assessing Global Injury—Injury Severity Score

Several objective indices have been developed to objectively quantify the acuity and prognosis in polytrauma. In 1974, Baker et al. developed the Injury Severity Score (ISS) for patients with disparate injury patterns from the existing Abbreviated Injury Scale (AIS) (10). They quantified the severity of injury to multiple systems in order to predict mortality. Using the AIS as a model, the head and neck, face, chest, abdominal or pelvic contents, extremities, pelvic girdle, and general health were evaluated on a 5-point severity scale. The scores of the three most severely injured areas were squared and added. An ISS of 10 or less predicted zero mortality, whereas a score of 50 or greater predicted a 100% death rate. Additional non-life-threatening injuries were found to increase mortality in patients with a life-threatening injury. Elderly patients have a significantly elevated mortality for all ISS scores. The ISS was more successful than the AIS at predicting mortality.

Since the inception of the landmark ISS, multiple scoring systems have evolved as numerical descriptors of injury severity and predictors of mortality (11–19). It is hoped that these statistical models may be used to evaluate both injury severity prospectively and the success of trauma care retrospectively. The success and limitations of each system has been evaluated in prospective and retrospective studies (20–27). Each model has been shown to enhance the prognostic capabilities of trauma scoring in specific populations; however, there is no consensus on the utility of a single scoring system that universally offers significant improvements over the ISS. Among orthopedic traumatologists, therefore, the ISS is used universally to communicate the severity of a patient's global injury.

2. Injury to a Single Extremity—Mangled Extremity Score

Treatment of a single limb with severe trauma involves the difficult question of salvage or amputation. Prolonged attempts to salvage a limb are costly, morbid, often ultimately ineffective, and at times lethal. The Mangled Extremity Severity Score (MESS) was created to predict when primary amputation of the lower extremity should be performed following major trauma (28,29). Lower extremity injuries with significant vascular compromise and open fracture were scored based on severity of skeletal and soft tissue injury, shock, ischemia, and patient age. A MESS of 7 or greater was 100% predictive of amputation in both retrospective and prospective analyses. Retrospective studies at level 1 trauma centers in the United States and United Kingdom have validated the MESS for severe lower extremity injuries (28–31). In an effort to quantify the risk of upper extremity injury, the MESS has been extrapolated to the upper limb in retrospective studies (32). A MESS of 7 or higher has been found to predict a decision to amputate the upper extremity. However, in deciding to amputate an upper extremity, the MESS is helpful but not absolute. The clinical judgment, technical skills, and experience of the operating surgeon must ultimately be taken into account. Upper extremity amputees are reluctant to use prosthetic devices, as these are cumbersome and provide inadequate function. This necessitates, in most cases, an attempt to salvage the upper limb. Since upper extremity amputation is lifestyle-altering, a second opinion in such scenarios is often helpful. In the setting of complex brachial plexus injuries, root avulsions, or axillary vessel injuries, however, the MESS objectively supports limb amputation and helps prevent unrealistic salvage attempts for a limb that will ultimately be nonviable or nonfunctioning (32).

3. Assessing Individual Upper Extremity Injuries

Within the context of the five phases of trauma management, the evaluation of individual injuries should take place once the primary survey ABCs are completed and the resuscitation is begun. Open fractures are classified using the Gustilo classification system (33,34), which aids in decision making regarding treatment.

1. Type I injuries are open fractures with wounds of less than 1 cm that usually occur as inside-out injuries when a bony spike punctures the overlying skin. The fragment often reduces spontaneously, leaving a small puncture hole as the only evidence of a much more significant injury. Contamination of the bone, however, is minimal. Type I injuries show no significant periosteal stripping and have a minimal soft tissue component.
2. Type II injuries are greater than 1 cm in size but involve minimal soft tissue compromise; it is usually possible to close these injuries primarily.
3. Type III injuries are of large size; they are further classified by their compounding injury component. Type IIIA involves massive contamination of a large soft tissue component, but soft tissue coverage is possible primarily, needing no flaps or grafts. Type IIIB indicates a wound that is significantly contaminated and will not close without a soft tissue transfer or flap. Gustilo type IIIC injuries include large open fractures with associated vascular injury that will require repair.

Fractures associated with blunt trauma without skin rents are often mistakenly considered less severe than open injuries. The lack of obvious injury to tissues other than bone is deceiving, and the threat of closed bony injuries is often minimized. Tscherne developed a soft tissue injury classification that aids physicians in communicating the severity of injuries associated with closed fractures (35):

1. Grade 0 includes trauma with negligible soft tissue injury.
2. Grade 1 includes minimal superficial abrasions and contusions overlying the fracture without a skin break.
3. Grade 2 injuries involve severe contusion at the injury site and contaminated abrasions. These injuries predict a significant compromise of the deep soft tissues.
4. Grade 3 injuries have an associated degloving component, vascular interruption, a crushing mechanism of injury, or threat of compartment syndrome.

The Tscherne classification alerts the orthopedic surgeon to the need for repeated reevaluation of the limb and soft tissues between a closed skin envelope and underlying fracture. It is a useful marker in the setting of upper extremity polytrauma, especially crush injuries and closed fractures due to high-energy impact. Unrecognized injuries that evolve after presentation are more likely to be identified if the injury in considered in this light.

Once an injury is identified, defined, and reduced, it should be splinted in a fashion that will allow reevaluation of the skin, soft tissues, any impending compartment syndrome, and neurological and vascular status. A baseline examination includes assessment of the pulses and capillary refill. Brachial, radial, and ulnar pulses must be examined. Allen's test defines the arterial supply distal to the wrist and tests the integrity of the radial artery–supplied deep palmar arch and the ulnar artery–fed superficial palmar arch. Doppler examination of arterial flow is necessary if pulses are not palpable. Duplex Doppler ultrasound of the deep venous system may be required if there is question of deep venous thrombosis or venous obstruction. If pulses cannot be confidently identified, angiography is imperative. In addition, if pulses are not present on initial evaluation, an assessment of the time since injury is necessary. This is useful in predicting the viability of the distal extremity, especially when viability of the distal remnant is uncertain and the risk of amputation is high. Ischemia time is of two varieties: cold ischemia time and warm ischemia time. Cold ischemia time is the time that passes while the limb is in ice, while warm ischemia time is the time when the limb is not in ice. Amputated extremities, once they are placed in plastic bags, are at risk of tissue damage because muscle depends on aerobic glycolysis for energy production. Therefore metabolites accumulate, including lactic acid, with sharp decrease in PH. After 2 h of ischemia, muscle can recover fairly readily. However, after 4 h, the recovery phase is rather prolonged; and after 6 h, recovery is unlikely. Replantation of an amputated limb proximal to the wrist is not supported with warm ischemia time greater than 6 h or cold ischemia time greater than 12 h. The more proximal the amputation, with requisite muscle mass, the less successful replantation because of ischemia, irreversible mitochondrial damage, and reperfusion injury (the reflow phenomenon).

A complete neurological examination is necessary on presentation. The presence or absence of sensation of pain and touch must be documented. The geographic margins of any deficit are then demarcated and annotated in the record. The integrity of the motor pathways must be tested for the cranial nerves and paraspinals and from the shoulder distally. Contraction of the deltoid indicates an intact axillary nerve. The musculocutaneous nerve innervates the biceps brachii, brachialis, and coracobrachialis; elbow flexion indicates an intact nerve. The triceps is supplied by the radial nerve. More distally, the radial nerve innervates the brachioradialis and wrist extensors. Ability to extend the fingers at the metacarpophalangeal (MP) joint indicates an intact posterior interosseous nerve, which is a branch of the radial nerve in the forearm. On the volar aspect of the forearm flexion at the wrist and finger flexion denote median nerve function. The anterior interosseous branch of the median nerve is tested with thumb interphalangeal and index distal interphalangeal flexion in pinch. Ulnar nerve motor function is tested with flexion of the two ulnar digits and abduction/adduction of the fingers.

The combination of sensory and motor nerve dysfunction should be identified and the possibility of a lesion at the brachial plexus or above must be considered. Therefore a complete understanding of the components of the deficits and of the upper extremity nervous system anatomy is critical. If a brachial plexus or spinal cord injury is suspected, then a complete central and autonomic nervous system evaluation is warranted. The presence of Horner's sign—ptosis, myosis, and anhydrosis—indicates injury to the sympathetic nerves proximal to the dorsal root ganglion. Not all of these signs may be present at the time of injury. It is important to determine the injury level, since postganglionic lesions can be grafted. While C5 to T1 may be injured independently by avulsion, isolated root lesions of C6 to C8 are unlikely. The deficit following truncal injuries are identical to those of root lesions (upper trunk C5 to C6, middle C8, lower C8 to T1). Thus it is not possible to differentiate between root and trunk injuries except when roots are damaged proximal to posterior primary rami, sympathetic rami, or motor nerves arising from roots directly. The trunks lie in the posterior triangle, where they are vulnerable to stab or gunshot wounds and traction injuries. During motor examination, the function of the rhomboids and serratus anterior should be carefully assessed. Paralyses of these muscles suggest a root avulsion, as the dorsal scapular and long thoracic nerves originate from the roots (C5 to 7). A positive Tinel's sign may evolve over 3 to 4 weeks, and this indicates a postganglionic injury. Shift of the head away from the injured side is evidence of denervation of the paraspinous muscles, strongly associated with root avulsion. Because sympathetic ganglion from T1–2 is close to the preganglionic fibers of T1 and C8, a Horner syndrome is strongly correlated with a C8 and/or T1 root avulsion. Modern techniques in imaging such as cervical myelography with or without a CT scan and magnetic resonance imaging (MRI or MR angiography for arterial/venous injuries) can confirm root lesions preoperatively. For example, CT myelography can visualize traumatic meningoceles (also called pseudomeningoceles), which correlate with avulsion of the corresponding root. However, false negatives and false positives exist with these new techniques.

Once the individual injuries are identified and the patient is stabilized, treatment of each component begins. The evolution of injuries throughout the stabilization, delayed operative procedures, and recovery phases must be monitored closely. Lack of progressive improvement during any one of these phases should alert the physician to a more complex injury than was determined or an unidentified injury. It is paramount to do a thorough neurovascular examination initially and repeat it often, looking for evolution of neurological injury. Good plain films of the cervical spine, shoulder girdle, and chest are complemented by CT and MRI of the spine and are useful in elucidating the etiology of the neural injury.

IV. PREVENTING ADDITIONAL POSTTRAUMATIC ILLNESS

In the resuscitation phase a patient commonly receives multiple units of blood products in order to preserve life and prevent shock. In this process it is not uncommon to create a coagulopathy through administration of products. The coagulopathy may simply be dilutional or due to inadequate replacement of clotting factors while repleting packed cells or fluid. A patient's reaction to blood products may also make the administered factors and platelets ineffective. The potential for this complication must be recognized; serial coagulation studies should be routinely used to monitor patients who receive multiple units of blood, platelets, and coagulation factors.

Deep venous thrombosis is associated with polytrauma due to the extensive period of immobilization that accompanies multiple-extremity injuries and their rehabilitation, pelvic fracture, and prolonged central nervous system depression. In the upper limb, axillary vein thrombosis, although rare, may be life- or limb-threatening and should be contemplated if there is massive limb swelling. The type of prophylaxis against this complication is not standardized, but its necessity is agreed upon. The authors' preferred method of anticoagulation is heparin 5000 u given subcutaneously twice daily (tailored to the patient's medical condition). The effect of this medication is terminated easily for repeated surgical procedures, and the medication is well tolerated.

A third common complication of traumatic injury that requires constant vigilance is compartment syndrome. This may occur as an effect of the primary injury, as part of the constellation of polytrauma, or as an iatrogenic injury associated with fracture treatment. Lack of recognition or delayed identification of compartment syndrome is a common cause of litigation related to trauma. Compartment syndrome is caused by the imbalance of arterial and venous flow, with resultant capillary shunting and muscle ischemia. The viability of all tissues within the compartment is at risk when the pressure rises above 30 mmHg or is within 10 to 30 mmHg of the diastolic pressure (for hypertensive or hypotensive patients). Common symptoms and signs of compartment syndrome include pain out of proportion to the injury, pallor, paresthesias, pulselessness, and paralysis; however, the earliest and most reliable sign is pain with passive stretch of tendons within the compartment. Diagnosis is confirmed with compartment pressure measurement, but signs and symptoms should guide the physician's urgent response when the clinical examination does not match complaints. When in doubt, serial compartment measurements should be performed. Treatment of the compartment syndrome involves surgical release of the individual compartments. The diagnosis of compartment syndrome is especially difficult to establish in patients with head injury or who are unconscious. In these patients, the orthopedic surgeon is guided more by physical findings, serial examinations of the firm compartment, vital signs indicating discomfort during testing, and objective measurements of compartment pressure either with serial measurements or with a continuous indwelling catheter. Early operative intervention is critical, as an untreated compartment syndrome will progress to tissue ischemia and necrosis, with resultant ischemic contracture and loss of function. Volar forearm compartment syndrome is common after high-energy trauma with or without skeletal injury. The deltoid muscle may also be individually affected. After fasciotomy, compartment signs often resolve.

The trauma patient, and especially the polytrauma patient, has special concerns related to the common types of injury sustained, the prolonged course of evaluation and treatment, and the types of medical intervention that must be addressed. Additional iatrogenic injury must be prevented through recognition of this potential and aggressive treatment once these common complications are recognized.

V. PRINCIPLES OF EARLY TRAUMA INTERVENTIONS

Therapeutic interventions in the traumatized patient are directed, upon presentation and until completion of care, toward minimizing the risk of complications and maximizing functional outcome. The traumatologist's plan of upper extremity care during the early phases of care must be aimed toward limb preservation, aggressive prophylaxis against infection, and continuous reevaluation of the degree of injury.

A sharp distinction between severe trauma to the upper and lower extremities is the importance of salvage measures of the mangled upper limb. Patients tolerate amputation of the upper extremity poorly. Salvage indications, therefore, are much broader for the upper extremity than the lower. Only the most mangled upper extremities are amputated acutely and, if so, fillet flaps are utilized to save a level of amputation, especially in the fingers. Prosthetic design has sought to overcome the resultant deficits of amputation by developing complex hinged devices with mechanical or motorized components. Patients, however, often find these prostheses cumbersome, ineffective at restoring function, and cosmetically unacceptable. They will usually not be worn when the contralateral limb is normal.

Tissue must demonstrate viability to merit salvage. Muscle may be evaluated based on its contractility, color, capacity to bleed, and consistency (36). Evidence of perfusion of other soft tissues, such as tendons and fat, cannot be so readily tested, and this lack will declare itself through necrosis. Although a patient may demonstrate nerve dysfunction on examination, the most common traumatic injury to nerves is contusion or stretch, and function usually returns. Consequently, identifiable nerves and their vascular beds should be preserved to allow adequate time for recovery, which may take several months.

High-energy injuries cause damage to soft tissues beyond the immediate vicinity of the wound; the zone of injury beyond the obvious must be determined. Surveillance of this boundary requires careful observation and follow-up, because ischemic tissue may not declare itself until several days after the injury. The importance of serial debridement to remove the necrotic tissue must be emphasized. Necrotic tissue not only increases the chance of local infection at the injury but also predisposes to the risk of systemic infection. Careful debridement, therefore, is of paramount importance.

Infection prophylaxis begins on presentation. After the initial examination of an open injury, the wound should be dressed with povidone-iodine (Betadine)–soaked sterile gauze and left with this dressing intact until the wound is reexamined in the OR at the time of initial irrigation and debridement. Irrigation and debridement either in the emergency room (ER) or OR should be as soon as the patient is seen or no later than 8 to 12 h from the time of injury. It is important to limit the inspection of wounds in the ER to decrease nosocomial contamination with resistant organisms.

Prophylactic antibiotics are administered immediately according to the Gustilo classification of open fractures. Gustilo I and II fractures should be treated with a first-generation cephalosporin. Gustilo IIIA fractures should be prophylaxed with a first-generation cephalosporin and an aminoglycoside. IIIB and IIIC fractures receive penicillin to cover streptococcal species. Open traumatic injuries are susceptible to tetanus infection. Tetanus prophylaxis, including tetanus toxoid and tetanus immune globulin, is indicated for injuries over 24 h old or when the patient has not received a booster within the preceding 5 years.

VI. EMERGENCY PROCEDURES

Operative treatment of open wounds begins with irrigation and debridement as soon as the patient is hemodynamically stable and when there are no other life-threatening injuries. Irrigation with high-pressure pulsatile lavage without admixed antibiotics significantly decreases the bacterial load at the wound. Wound debridement is based on the following principles:

1. Remove all debris.
2. Tangentially excise the wound margin.
3. Excise muscle that is nonviable.
4. Preserve nerve and blood supply.
5. Remove devitalized bone fragments.
6. Minimize damage to the joint capsule.
7. Anticipate multiple debridements and aggressively debride marginally viable tissue.
8. Do not primarily bone graft grade II and III injuries, even if skin closure can be performed.

Sharp debridement begins at the periphery of the wound and proceeds centrally. Viable skin and dermis demonstrates rapid capillary refill. All wounds require an aggressive investigation of the depth and extent of the injury. Skin rents are extended longitudinally to allow adequate exposure of the underlying muscle and periosteal contamination and to ensure complete decontamination of the soft tissue tracts caused by bony protrusion. Care must be taken not to disrupt the often marginal remaining blood supply to comminuted bone fragments. The margins of injured muscle and bone should be incised with a scalpel or curretted as part of the decontamination and debridement. Displaced tissues with intact arterial supply are then returned to their anatomic location. Loose fragments of bone are removed, since necrotic bone serves as a nidus for infection.

At the conclusion of the initial debridement, Gustilo type I fractures may be closed primarily. The decision to close a type II injury is based on clinical examination after irrigation and debridement are complete. Wound edges are approximated loosely with interrupted nonabsorbable suture; the use of deep absorbable and braided suture should be minimized. Any longitudinal extensions made for debriding the soft tissue of grade II and III injuries may be closed. Due to continued intraoperative swelling, however, this may be impossible. The surgeon may also prefer to leave these incisions open if continued swelling is anticipated. With serial debridements, the skin edges may meet as edema decreases. These extensions may then be closed. The use of relaxing incisions is decried, as this increased dissection of the fasciocutaneous plane may increase wound necrosis.

Open wounds are dressed to minimize contamination between serial debridements and until soft tissue coverage is accomplished. The type of dressing applied depends on the wound base and the goals of dressing changes. Dressings are therapeutic in their ability to decontaminate and encourage neovascularization. Wet-to-dry dressing changes with half-strength Dakin's solution aids in the decontamination of subacute infection and in the debridement of nonviable tissue with dressing removal. Vacuum-assisted dressings, such as the KCI Wound-Vac, are believed to incite microvascular ingrowth, thereby increasing the host defense against local infection and improving granulation of the wound bed. Also, semipermeable membranes allow transudate to egress while limiting bacterial access to the wound.

The goal of debridement is to identify the extent of injury, eliminate contamination, and preserve tissue that displays viability. Debridements are carried out at 24-to 72-h intervals, when the wound appears to be acutely infected, when the patient demonstrates new systemic evidence of infection without an identifiable source, or when demarcation necrosis is well established. When the wound margins show no additional evidence of ischemia and there is a viable vascular bed at the base of the wound, soft tissue reconstruction and coverage should be contemplated. Soft tissue coverage is the ultimate stage in preventing wound contamination and infection.

VII. DELAYED OPERATIVE PROCEDURES

Serial debridement of wounds helps minimize the risk of infection; however, the best prophylaxis is soft tissue coverage. Such coverage of complex open fractures is rarely a problem in the upper extremity unless the wounding force is extreme or degloving injury has occurred. However these injuries, when present, are often associated with loss of tendon, nerve, and artery; thus procedures for wound closures as well as repair or reconstruction of the injured tendon, nerve, or artery are required. Reconstruction should address all or maximum deficits at first surgery if feasible. If the debridement is adequate, reconstruction can be performed immediately. This may include rotation flaps outside the zone of injury that provide supple soft tissue coverage. Soft tissue reconstruction should also consider the esthetic appearance of the upper extremity. If healthy granulation tissue or viable muscle is present following serial debridements, split thickness skin grafting from remote sites is optimal. For wounds needing thicker dermis with less contraction, a full-thickness graft is a preferred option. Meshing of a split-thickness graft allows efflux of the edema and blood and coverage of a wider area. The graft contracts as the wound heals, which leaves behind a smaller scar.

For small full-thickness defects, rotational flaps from within the upper extremity provide adequate blood supply and coverage (Fig. 1). For some injuries, myocutaneous rotational flaps in the upper extremity are limited, as mobilization of one or more muscular components can significantly impair the patient's postoperative function. That is why fasciocutaneous flaps are preferred. There are a number of island pedicle flaps available for the hand. These are the reversed radial artery forearm flap, posterior interosseous flap, ulnar forearm flap, radial or ulnar perforator flaps, etc. The groin flap is another option but has the drawbacks of restricting the extremity, requiring a second surgery for division, and keeping the limb in a dependent position. In massive defects, a free flap must be considered. For the forearm, the latissimus dorsi is used as an island pedicle flap to the elbow. For areas distally, the latissimus must be taken as a free flap. Wounds over the elbow and humerus are usually treated with skin grafting, pedicled latissimus flap, and proximally based radial artery forearm flap. The pedicled latissimus flap can be harvested as a muscle or myocutaneous flap. Innervated flaps, like the gracilis, provide power and coverage and animate the hand. Also, free flaps have allowed savalge of the upper extremity and have permitted tendon grafting over the dorsum of the degloved, burned, or crushed hand. The advancement of free tissue transfer has significantly augmented the salvage measures of open fractures and enhanced the indications for upper extremity preservation at trauma centers where plastic surgery and hand specialists are integrated into the trauma team.

VIII. PRINCIPLES OF OPEN UPPER EXTREMITY FRACTURE FIXATION

Early internal fixation of Gustilo I, II, and IIIA to C open upper extremity fractures results in acceptable postoperative function and union and has a limited incidence of infection (37–43). Definitive treatment should be performed as early as possible and should not be delayed for repeated irrigation and debridement. Primary fixation helps preserve the integrity of the overlying soft tissues, restores the periosteal and endosteal blood supplies, and allows early healing at the fracture site. When a fracture is fixed acutely with hardware, metal should not be left exposed to dressings or the environment because this increases the risk of infection. Closure or flap coverage of these wounds follows at an appropriate interval on a case-by-case basis, usually within several days to a week, to lower the incidence of osteomyelitis.

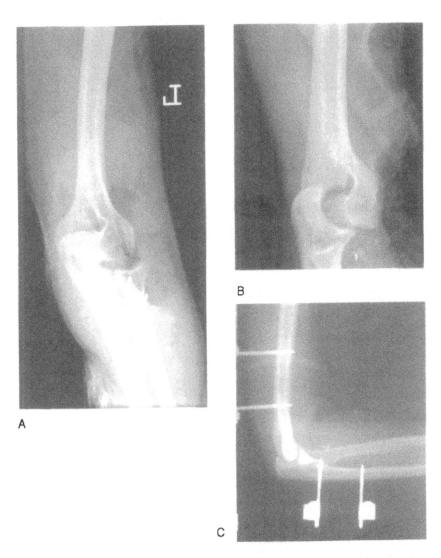

Figure 1   A and B. Grade 3C open fracture/dislocation and lateral degloving injury to the left elbow sustained in a single car rollover MVA. The brachial artery, median nerve, and radial nerve were disrupted. C. Initial treatment consisted of spanning external fixation of the elbow fracture/dislocation to allow soft tissue reconstruction. Vein graft reconstruction of the brachial artery was performed (vascular clips present on x-ray).

The success rate of primary open reduction and internal fixation of open upper extremity fractures has limited the indications for external fixation. As a result, the indications for external fixation have decreased significantly. Gustilo IIIC injuries and injuries with significant neurological injury have been treated with monolateral external fixators (44–47). In these salvage operations, external fixation may be an integral step in the primary reconstruction of the limb's neu-

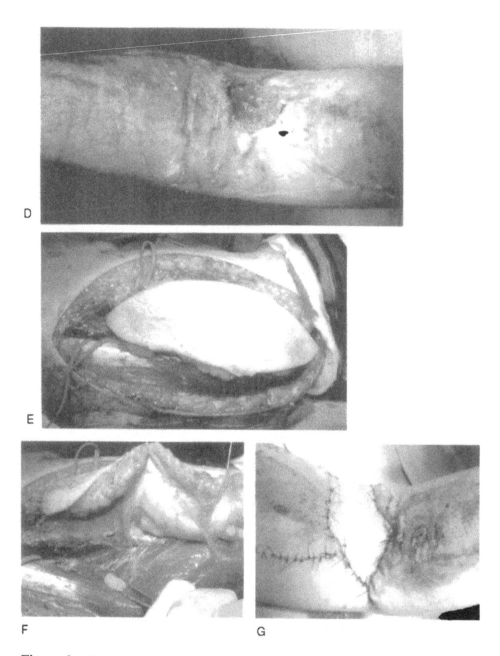

Figure 1 Continued. D. Early cicatrix formation produced a nonmobile soft tissue envelope that compromised further reconstructive efforts. E. Reconstruction required the mobilization of soft tissues and creation of a mobile soft tissue bed for vein grafting. A pedicled fasciocutaneous lateral arm flap was raised and rotated into the antecubital fossa. This allowed staged reconstruction of artery and nerves. F. Fasciocutaneous vessels of the lateral arm flap. G. Flap coverage protects neurovascular structures and allows motion at the elbow.

rovascular supply. Usually this is a temporizing measure, especially around open and unstable elbow fracture/dislocations. Additionally, the external fixator facilitates the multitudinous operations that are inherent to this severity of upper extremity injury, including delayed bone grafting, soft tissue reconstruction, and free tissue transfer. One common use is for extreme comminution and instability of the metaphyseal fractures of the distal radius, which are effectively treated with spanning external fixation.

Although external fixation has clear advantages, there are multiple inherent disadvantages that limit its use in definitive treatment of fractures. Decreased elbow motion, significant rates of malunion and nonunion, and pin-tract infection plague this treatment method. The rate of nonunion associated with external fixation of open upper extremity fracture is reported to be 6% (48). The use of external fixation as a primary treatment of explosive wartime injuries of the upper extremity is associated with a 20% rate of nonunion (48) and 17% rate of malunion (45). Nearly 50% patients have pin-tract infection (44,45), while 3 to 10% develop osteomyelitis (46,48). Stiffness of the elbow is ubiquitous following external fixation of the upper extremity. For periarticular and intraarticular injuries, external fixators must cross the elbow, which delays postoperative physical therapy and causes significant elbow stiffness. Other complications, such as nerve injury from pin placement and fracture through pinholes, have also been reported.

External fixation is useful in a very limited number of severely traumatized upper extremity injuries including those with tenuous neurovascular status and massively comminuted fractures with or without segmental bone loss. It quickly creates a stable environment for vascular repair and allows access to the wound for multiple debridements. Due to the complications of this treatment, however, its role is limited and the fixator should be removed at the earliest opportunity to minimize postoperative deficits.

IX. DEFINITIVE TREATMENT OF UPPER-EXTREMITY FRACTURE PATTERNS

Certain fractures of the upper extremity merit inclusion in any discussion of upper extremity polytrauma and open fractures since their incidence is increased in this setting. These include fractures of the proximal humerus, humeral shaft, and distal humerus; open fracture and fracture/dislocation at the elbow, and diaphyseal fractures of the forearm.

A. The Humerus

Fractures of the humerus are described as proximal humeral fractures (including fracture/dislocations of the glenohumeral joint), shaft fractures (described as proximal, middle, and distal third), and distal humeral fractures (including intraarticular fractures).

1. Proximal Humeral Fractures

Evaluation of fractures of the proximal humerus relies on the identification of the four main fracture fragments: the articular surface, the greater and lesser tuberosities, and the shaft. Knowledge of the muscular attachments of each of these fragments allows the surgeon to predict the displacement pattern. Due to the insertion of the supraspinatus tendon on the greater tuberosity, the fragment usually displaces posteriorly and superiorly. The lesser tuberosity generally displaces medially and superiorly while the lastisimus dorsi and pectoralis major muscles pull medially on the proximal shaft of the humerus. The blood supply to the proximal humerus consists of the anterior and posterior circumflex arteries, which are branches of the distal axillary artery given at the level of the subscapularis muscle. The main nutrient artery is the arcuate artery of Liang, a branch of the ascending branch of the anterior circumflex humeral artery. Displacement of the lesser tuberosity, where this artery lies, suggests that significant disruption of the vascular supply to the proximal humerus has occurred.

Dislocation of the glenohumeral joint is usually diagnosed by history and then confirmed on orthogonal radiographs. A trauma series (anteroposterior, lateral, and axillary views) demonstrates the dislocated head. Often the axillary x-ray is most helpful in making the diagnosis. A Velpeau axillary view may always be performed, regardless of the injury type. The presence or absence of a Bankart or Hill-Sachs lesion should be determined prior to any reduction move and should be documented. Dislocation of the glenohumeral joint should be reduced emergently in the ER except if severe fracture/dislocation is suspected. Early reduction restores bony alignment and minimizes further neurological and vascular compromise to the upper extremity. Glenohumeral dislocation without a compounding fracture is treated in a sling with close follow-up. The duration of sling wear is debatable and is based on the patient's age and level of activity, the presence of associated injury, and the patient's history of prior dislocation. The authors prefer to limit reduction attempts to three in the ER before taking the patient to the OR for closed reduction under general anesthesia.

Fractures of the proximal humerus are described by the Neer classification (49). Fracture fragments of the proximal humerus include the articular surface, the diaphysis, and the two tuberosities. The classification varies from undisplaced fracture pattern to a four-part fracture with displacement. Significant parts are those that are displaced 5 mm or angulated 45 degrees. This fracture classification system is based on the likelihood of vascular disruption and the risk of osteonecrosis of the fracture fragments, which is directly proportional to the number of displaced parts. CT evaluation is often necessary to fully evaluate complex fracture patterns, discern the involvement of the articular surface, and measure the displacement of each fragment.

Treatment options are selected based on the number of significant fracture parts. Two-part fractures of the surgical neck are usually treated with closed management. In the rare case of open two-part fracture, open reduction and internal fixation (ORIF) with suture or wire tension band, with or without Enders rods, may be employed following irrigation and debridement. Two part fracture of the greater tuberosity is an indication for operative reduction and fixation because of the risk of impingement with nonoperative therapy. This may be accomplished through a limited approach and suture fixation, tension-band wiring, or screw fixation. Interest has reemerged in percutaneous pinning of unstable two-part fractures. The results of this treatment depend on the surgeon's ability to reduce the fracture anatomically.

Three- and four-part fractures of the proximal humerus have been treated with success utilizing multiple internal fixation methods. Suture fixation, periarticular plates, and blade plates offer multiple points of fixation for fracture fragments. Newer locking plates make the plate-screw construct a fixed-angle device. Periosteal stripping during ORIF of three- or four-part fractures leads to increased risk of avascular necrosis (AVN) of the head. The risk of AVN in three-part fractures treated with ORIF is 27% (50). Since the vascular supply to the humeral head ascends adjacent to the lesser tuberosity, displaced fracture of the lesser tuberosity imposes a higher risk of AVN. Nonunion, malunion, postoperative infection, poor functional outcome, and hardware impingement also complicate internal fixation methods. The results of salvage humeral head replacement for failed ORIF of three- and four-part fractures have been reported to be significantly worse than the primary hemiarthroplasty (51). The orthopedic surgeon must have alternative fixation devices and humeral head prostheses readily available when primary fixation is elected. The decision to convert to humeral head replacement is made intraoperatively and helps preserve the vascularity of the tuberosities.

Four-part fracture of the humeral head, head-splitting fractures, and anatomical neck fractures are indications for humeral hemiarthroplasty. Primary hemiarthroplasty can predictably alleviate pain. The patient should be cautioned, however, that the range of motion of this limb will be limited.

2. Diaphyseal Humeral Fractures

The close proximity of many neurological and vascular structures to the humeral shaft puts these structures at high risk for concurrent injury. In particular, spiral distal-third diaphyseal fractures—i.e., Holstein-Lewis fractures—are associated with a high incidence of radial nerve injury because of the relative immobility of the radial nerve as it pierces the lateral intermuscular septum (52).

Treatment of shaft fractures is directed by fracture angulation and displacement as well as compounding factors such as open fracture, associated fractures, and neurovascular injury. Patients tolerate up to 30 degrees of varus/valgus angulation, 20 degrees of sagittal malalignment, 2 cm of shortening, and 15 degrees of malrotation. Most closed injuries can be treated nonoperatively. Open fracture and polytrauma are both indications for surgical management of fractures of the humeral diaphysis (Fig. 2). Floating elbow injuries, bilateral humeral diaphysis fractures, segmental fracture, and polytrauma to both upper and lower extremities

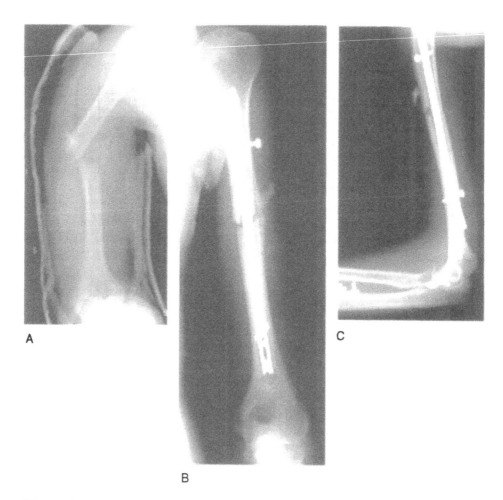

A

B

C

Figure 2 A. Diaphyseal humeral fracture sustained by a pedestrian who was struck by a truck. The patient sustained an ipsilateral tibial plateau fracture and multiple system injuries. At the level of the fracture, the arm was massively swollen, indicating severe disruption of the soft tissues despite intact skin. B and C. Locked retrograde intramedullary nailing of the humerus was indicated due to ipsilateral extremity injuries and polytrauma.

also are absolute indications. Postreduction radial nerve palsy, a large body habitus, and pathological fracture are relative indications for operative nerve exploration and fracture treatment.

Internal fixation of the diaphyseal humerus is limited to ORIF with compression plating or intramedullary fixation. Among fixation devices the 4.5-mm dynamic compression plate (DCP) is considered the "gold standard" for diaphyseal humeral fractures. Eight cortices above and below the fracture site are required for optimal fixation. The 4.5-mm plate provides multiaxial screw fixation and supplants the 3.5-mm DCP due to smaller plate's inability to provide rota-

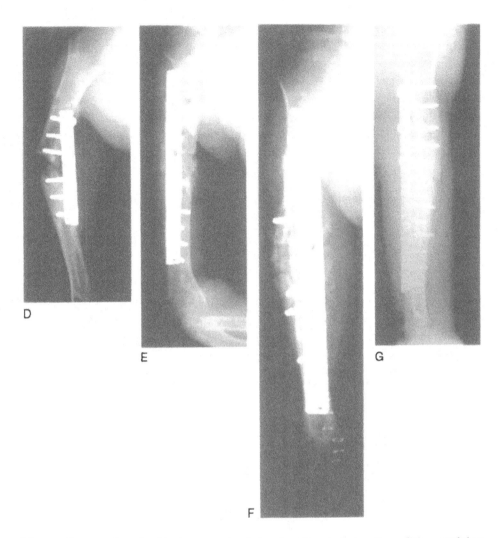

Figure 2 Continued. D. As a result of the significant destruction of the overlying soft tissues, the transverse fracture went on to nonunion. Initial attempts at open plating were inadequate secondary to insufficient plate length. E to G. Ultimately the fracture required longer plate fixation and combined autograft and allograft to unite.

tional stability. Some smaller humeri, however, can effectively be treated with the 3.5-mm DCP plate. During humeral plating, using the posterior approach, the radial nerve must be identified and protected throughout reduction and fixation. Humeral shaft plating yields an overall union rate of 96%, with an incidence of radial nerve palsy of 2% (53).

Both antegrade and retrograde humeral nailing have recently gained increasing popularity due to their limited exposure, indirect reduction techniques, and stability. Disadvantages include prominent proximal hardware and rotator cuff injury with proximally inserted nails and elbow stiffness and distal humeral fracture with retrograde nails. Humeral nails are indicated in proximal and middle-third fractures, segmental fractures, and some distal fractures. The proximity of neurovascular structures to the fracture site argues against reaming. Static locking of the nail is recommended. The nonunion rate for humeral nailing varies from 0 to 29%, while shoulder pain or stiffness varies from 5 to 27%. The utility of nailing for acute open fracture, with or without reaming, has yet to gain the support that tibial nailing has achieved among traumatologists.

3. Distal Humeral Fractures

The complex geometry of the distal humerus makes treatment of these fractures especially difficult. Two columns comprise the distal humerus. The lateral column terminates in the capitellar articulation and the medial column forms the trochlea distally. There is little osseous support between these two columns. Coursing around the distal humerus from posterolaterally at the lateral intermuscular septum to anteriorly at the anterior capsule, the radial nerve is in close proximity to distal humerus fractures. The ulnar nerve is also at high risk of injury in the ulnar groove medial to the trochlea. Identification of these structures is imperative in the operative management of distal humeral fractures.

Distal humeral fractures are classified according to their geometry. They are described as one- or two-column fractures and further by their radiographic appearance. The letters T, Y, H, and λ (lambda) are used as descriptors of different common patterns.

Comminuted distal-third and intraarticular T and Y condylar humeral fractures should universally be treated with rigid plate fixation. Biomechanical data most strongly support open reduction and internal fixation of both columns of the distal humerus using two plates oriented at 90 degrees to each other. A 3.5-mm DCP is contoured to the posterior aspect of the lateral column, wrapping distally up to the capitellar articular surface. A medial 3.5-mm DCP or pelvic reconstruction plate is used with screws, preferably in the coronal plane. This allows fixation through the axis of the trochlea at right angles to the lateral column fixation. Alternatively, a posterior plate on the medial column with sagitally oriented screws provides stable osteosynthesis. There are some new contoured periarticular plates that may help in reconstructing highly comminuted fractures. There is no substitute for 90 to 90 degree plating in internal fixation of a comminuted distal humerus. Very poor osteoporotic bone that fails to hold internal fixation when tested in the operating room may require primary total elbow arthroplasty in very limited circumstances.

B. The Elbow: Fracture/Dislocation of the Elbow

Most fracture/dislocations of the elbow are unstable and need ORIF. Dislocations are commonly posterior and are often associated with fractures of radial head, neck and coronoid and soft tissue injuries. Medial epicondylar avulsion is common in adolescents and is a result of associated valgus stress.

Injury to the brachial artery is rare but may range from intimal tear to transection. Arteriography must be done in the OR before reconstruction with a saphenous vein graft is attempted. Arterial thrombosis can lead to delayed occlusion and usually follows intimal tears. As this evolves gradually, monitoring is a must. Dislocation can injure median, ulnar, and anterior interosseous nerves. The majority of nerve injuries are neuropraxic; exploration is indicated only if the nerve fails to recover by 3 to 4 months.

During ORIF, coronoid fracture fixation is very important for the stability of the elbow. Radial head excision without replacement with prosthetic head is contraindicated in the presence of a coronoid fracture. ORIF of the radial head

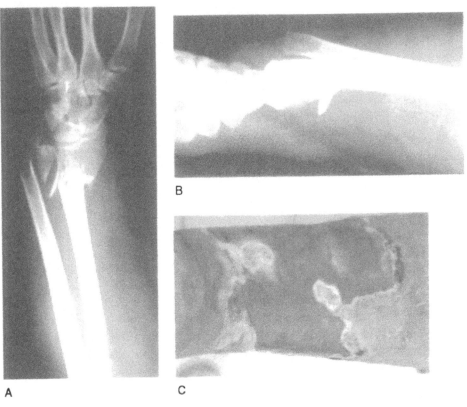

A   C

Figure 3 A and B. Violent open both bone-fracture of the distal forearm sustained in an MVA. Extensive comminution was present at the distal radius. C and D. The circumferential soft tissue injury was treated with splinting and staged debridements until the zone of the injury was completely demarcated. This ringer injury compromised exposure and mandated early definitive treatment. E and F. Radical escharectomy, split-thickness skin grafting, and definitive fixation were performed as staged procedures. Extensive radial comminution required compensatory ulnar shortening. Radial plating of the distal radius provides rigid stability.

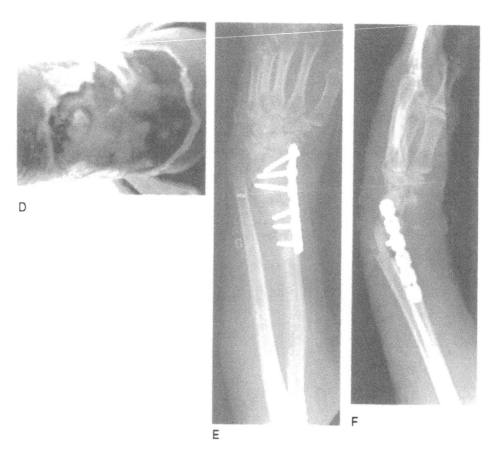

D

E

F

Figure 3 Continued.

is preferable if the head is salvageable. If not, a metallic head implant is substituted and the lateral collateral ligament complex is repaired.

Stiffness and posttraumatic arthritis are common and frustrating complications of elbow fracture/dislocation. Heterotopic ossification is common and can cause total ankylosis. Its severity is proportional to the severity of injury, latent subluxation, and length of immobilization. Indomethacin and radiation therapy are modalities to prevent or minimize this complication.

C. The Forearm

Although open fractures of the radius and ulna are obvious, it is still possible to miss a type I injury if the entire circumference is not inspected. This is especially true if the patient is unconscious or unable to provide an adequate history and is more common for distal metaphyseal both-bone forearm fractures. High-velocity gunshot injuries with cavitation effect, especially, are associated with neurovascular damage and must be explored carefully. Determination of the depth of the open wound and its proper assessment is best carried out in the operating room in sterile surroundings. Extensive debridement followed by primary ORIF or, in rare instances, external fixation is recommended. An external fixator is indicated in patients with soft tissue loss, bone loss (for maintaining length), associated open elbow fracture/dislocations, and severely contaminated wounds. Otherwise primary ORIF is the treatment of choice for open radius and ulnar fractures (Fig. 3). Early soft tissue reconstruction has much lower infection rate and lower flap failure rate; it is preferred over later reconstruction.

X. CONCLUSIONS

The treatment of polytrauma and open fractures of the upper extremity begins with standardized life- and limb- preserving protocols. Specific injury patterns determine how these protocols are utilized for individual patients with multisystem and multiple-extremity trauma. Staged treatment of complex injuries promotes the most rapid reconstructive opportunities and the earliest and most optimal return of function. Following the established principles of debridement, staged operations, fixation, soft tissue coverage, and rehabilitation directs efficient care.

The limitations of upper extremity prosthetics and the evolution of soft tissue and bony reconstruction have encouraged surgeons to attempt limb salvage in many cases. The ISS and MESS help the experienced surgeon make the rare decision to amputate the upper extremity. External fixation, when used, usually provides temporary stabilization until definitive reconstruction becomes feasible. Immediate fixation and treatment of these injuries, however, is leading to improved outcomes without increased risk of long-term complications.

REFERENCES

1. MC Henry, JE Hollander, JM Alicandro, G Cassara, S O'Malley, HC Thode Jr. Prospective countywide evaluation of the effects of motor vehicle safety device use on hospital resource use and injury severity. Ann Emerg Med 28(6):709–710, 1996.
2. RA Retting, BN Persaud, PE Garder, D Lord. Crash and injury reduction following installation of roundabouts in the United States. Am J Public Health 91(4):628–631, 2001.
3. A Lerner, S Stahl, H Stein. Hybrid external fixation in high-energy elbow fractures: A modular system with a promising future. J Trauma 49(6): 1017–1022, 2000.
4. G Wolff, M Dittman, T Reudi. Koordination von Chirurge und Intensivmedizin zur Vermeidung der posttraumatischen respiratorischen Insuffizienz. Unfallheilkunde 81:425–442, 1978.
5. G Teasdale, B Jennett. Assessment of coma and impaired consciousness: A practical scale. Lancet 2:81–84, 1974.
6. LB Bone, LB, K McNamara, B Shine. Mortality in multiple trauma patients with fractures. J Trauma 37: 262–265, 1994.
7. PL Broos, KH Stappaerts, EJ Luiten. The importance of early internal fixation in multiply injured patients to prevent late death due to sepsis. Injury 18:235–237, 1987.

8.   KD Johnson, A Cadambi, GB Seibert. Incidence of adult respiratory distress syndrome in patients with multiple musculoskeletal injuries: Effect of early operative stabilization of fractures. J Trauma 25: 375–384, 1985.

9.   R Seibel, J LaDuca, JM Hasset. Blunt multiple trauma, femur traction, and the pulmonary failure-septic state. Ann Surg 202: 283–295, 1985.

10. SP Baker, B O'Neill, W Haddon, WB Long. The injury severity score: A method for describing patients with multiple injuries and evaluating emergency care. J Trauma 14(3):187–196, 1974.

11. DA Kuhls, DL Malone, RJ McCarter, LM Napolitano. Predictors of mortality in adult trauma patients: The physiologic trauma score is equivalent to the Trauma and Injury Severity Score. J Am Coll Surg 194(6):695–704, 2002.

12. T Osler, SP Baker, W Long. A modification of the Injury Severity Score that both improves accuracy and simplifies scoring. J Trauma 43(6):922–925, 1997.

13. T Osler, R Rutledge, J Deis, E Bedrick. ICISS: An international classification of Disease-9 based Injury Severity Score. J Trauma 41(3):380–387, 1996.

14. CR Boyd, MA Tolson, WS Copes. Evaluating trauma care: The TRISS methodology. J Trauma 27:370–378, 1987.

15. WA Knaus, EA Draper, DP Wagner, JE Zimmerman. APACHE II: A severity of disease classification system. Crit Care Med 13:818–829, 1985.

16. WA Knaus, DP Wagner, EA Draper, et al. The APACHE III prognostic system: Risk prediction of hospital mortality for critically ill hospitalized adults. Chest 100: 1619–1636, 1991.

17. MJ Vassar, CL Wilkerson, PJ Duran, CA Perry, JW Holcroft. Comparison of APACHE II, TRISS, and a proposed 24-hour ICU point system for prediction of outcome in ICU trauma patients. J Trauma 32:490–499, 1992.

18. HR Champion, WJ Sacco, AJ Carnazzo, et al. Trauma score. Crit Care Med 9:672, 1981.

19. HR Champion, WS Copes, WJ Sacco. A revision of the Trauma Score. J Trauma 29:623–629, 1989.

20. R Rutledge. The Injury Severity Score is unable to differentiate between poor care and severe injury. J Trauma 40(6):944–950, 1996.

21. R Rutledge, DB Hoyt, AB Eastman, MJ Sise, T Velky, T Canty, T Wachtel, TM Osler. Comparison of the Injury Severity Score and ICD-9 Diagnosis Codes as predictors of outcome in injury: Analysis of 44,032 patients. J Trauma 42(3):477–487, 1997.

22. R Rutledge, T Osler, S Emery, S Kromhout-Schiro. The end of the Injury Severity Score (ISS) and the Trauma and Injury Severity Score (TRISS): ICISS, an International Classification of Diseases, ninth revision–based prediction tool, outperforms both ISS and TRISS as predictors of trauma patient survival, hospital charges, and hospital length of stay. J Trauma 44(1):41–48, 1998.

23. EL Hannan, L Szupulski Farrell, SFH Gorthy, PQ Bessey, CG Cayten, A Cooper, L Mottley. Predictors of mortality in adult patients with blunt injuries in New York state: a comparison of the Trauma and Injury Severity Score (TRISS) and the International Classification of Disease, ninth revision–based Injury Severity Score (ICISS). J Trauma 47(1):8–13, 1999.

24. GV Poole, M Tinsley, AK Tsao, KR Thomae, RW Martin, CJ Hauser. Abbreviated Injury Scale does not reflect the added morbidity of multiple lower extremity fractures. J Trauma 40(6):951–954, 1996.

25. E Grisoni, A Stallion, ML Nance, JL Lelli Jr, VF Garcia, E Marsh. The New Injury Severity Score and the evaluation of pediatric trauma. J Trauma 50(6):1006–1110, 2001.

26. HR Champion, WS Copes, WJ Sacco, CF Frey, JW Holcroft, DB Hoyt, JA Weigelt. Improved predictions from A Severity Characterization of Trauma (ASCOT) over Trauma and Injury Severity Score (TRISS): Results of an independent evaluation. J Trauma 40(1):40–48, 1996.

27. MJ Vassar, FR Lewis Jr, JA Chambers, RJ Mullins, PE O'Brien, JA Weigelt, MTR Hoang, JW Holcroft. Prediction of outcome in intensive care unit trauma patients: a multicenter study of Acute Physiology and Chronic Health Evaluation (APACHE), Trauma and Injury Severity Score (TRISS), and a 24-hour Intensive Care Unit Point System. J Trauma 47(2):324–329, 1999.

28. K Johansen, M Daines, T Howley, et al. Objective criteria accurately predict amputation following lower extremity trauma. J Trauma 30:568–573, 1990.

29. DL Helfet, T Howey, R Sanders, K Johansen. Limb salvage versus amputation. Preliminary results of the Mangled Extremity Score. Clin Orthop 256:80–86, 1990.

30. MG McNamara, JD Heckman, FG Corley. Severe open fractures of the lower extremity: A retrospective analysis of the Mangled Extremity Score (MESS). J Orthop Trauma 8:81–87, 1994.

31. PA Robertson. Prediction of amputation after severe lower limb trauma. J Bone Joint Surg Br 73-B:816–818, 1991.

32. JR Slauterbeck, C Britton, MS Moneim, FW Clevenger. Mangled extremity severity score: An accurate guide to treatment of the severely injured upper extremity. J Orthop Trauma 8(4):282–285, 1994.

33. RB Gustilo, J Anderson. Prevention of infection in the treatment of one thousand and twenty-five open fractures of long bones. J Bone Joint Surg 58-A(4):453–58, 1976.

34. RB Gustilo, RM Mendoza, DN Williams. Problems in the management of type III (severe) open fractures: A new classification of type III open fractures. J Trauma 24:742–746, 1984.

35. H Tscherne, G Regel, HC Pape, T Pohlemann, C Krettek. Internal fixation of multiple fractures in patients with polytrauma. Clin Orthop 347:62–78, 1998.

36. RE Sculley, CP Artz, Y Sako. An evaluation of the surgeon's criteria for determining the viability of muscle during debridement. Arch Surg 73:1031–1035, 1956.

37. BR Moed, JF Kellam, RJ Foster. Immediate internal fixation of open fractures of the diaphysis of the forearm. J Bone Joint Surg 68-A(7):1008–1017, 1986.

38. JA Jones. Immediate internal fixation of high-energy open forearm fractures. J Orthop Trauma 5(3):272–279, 1991.

39. K Yokoyama, M Shindo, M Itoman, M Yamamoto, N Sasamoto. Immediate internal fixation for open fractures of the long bones of the upper and lower extremities. J Trauma 37(2):230–236, 1994.

40. RB Gustilo. Current concepts in the management of open fractures. AAOS Instructional Course Lectures 36:359, 1987.

41. RB Gustilo, RP Gruninger, T Davis. Classification of type III (severe) open fracture relative to treatment and results. Orthopedics 10(12):1781, 1987.

42. JJ Wild, GW Hanson, JB Bennett, et al. External fixation use in the management of massive upper extremity trauma. Clin Orthop 164:172, 1982.

43. MD Putnam, TM Walsh. External fixation for open fractures of the upper extremity. Hand Clin 9(4):613–623, 1993.

44. LS Levin, RD Goldner, JR Urbaniak, JA Nunley, WT Hardaker. Management of severe musculoskeletal injuries of the upper extremity. J Orthop Trauma 4(4):432–440, 1990.

45. HR Mostafavi, P Tornetta. Open fractures of the humerus treated with external fixation. Clin Orthop 337:187–197, 1997.

46. DK Smith, WP Cooney. External fixation of high- energy upper extremity injuries. J Orthop Trauma 4(1):7–18, 1990.

47. RRR Hammer, B Rooser, D Lidman, S Smeds. Simplified external fixation for primary management of severe musculoskeletal injuries under war and peacetime conditions. J Orthop Trauma 10(8):545–554, 1996.

48. B Has, S Jovanovic, B Wertheimer, I Mikolasevic, P Grdic. External fixation as a primary and definitive treatment of open limb fractures. Injury 26(4):245–248, 1995.

49. CS Neer. Displaced proximal humerus fractures: part I—Classification and evaluation. J Bone Joint Surg 52A:1090–1103, 1970.

50. P Schai, A Imhoff, S Preiss. Comminuted humeral head fractures: A multicenter analysis. J Shoulder Elbow Surg 4(5):319–330, 1995.

51. RT Goldman, KJ Koval, F Cuomo. Functional outcomes after humeral head replacement for acute three- and four-part proximal humerus fractures. J Shoulder Elbow Surg 4:81, 1995.

52. A Holstein, GB Lewis. Fractures of the humerus with radial nerve paralysis. J Bone Joint Surg Am 45:1382–1388, 1963.

53. LA Hartsock. Humeral shaft fractures. In: Kellam JF, ed. Orthopaedic Knowledge Update Trauma II. Rosemont, Illinois: Amer Acad Ortho Surg, 2000.

8

Surgical Approaches to Upper Extremity Trauma

Carlos Mario Olarte
Hospital de San José, Fundación Universitaria de Ciencias de la Salud,
Bogotá, Colombia

Rodrigo Pesantez
Fundación Santa Fe de Bogotá, Universidad del Rosario,
Bogotá, Colombia

One of the most important things in trauma surgery is the preoperative planning of the surgery and above all the selection of the surgical approach. This chapter reviews the most common surgical approaches for upper extremity trauma, starting in the shoulder and finishing in the forearm. In each one of these instances, the indications, position of the patient, incision, and surgical dissection are reviewed. The shoulder is included as a brief section since in some cases of humeral fracture a more proximal extensile exposure may be required.

I. SURGICAL EXTENSIONS OF HUMERAL APPROACHES TO THE SHOULDER

A. Anterior Approach—Deltopectoral Approach

1. Incision

As an extension of the approach to the anterior, lateral, or medial approach to the humerus, the more distal incision head to the more standard deltopectoral incision.

2. Surgical Dissection

The internervous plane is located between the deltoid, the axillary nerve, and the pectoralis major, medial, and lateral pectoral nerves.

Once you incise the skin, you will find the cephalic vein in the deltopectoral groove, with the deltoid laterally and the pectoralis major medially. Take care to preserve the vein, do the dissection with your fingers, and take the vein with the deltoid laterally and the pectoralis major medially.

Then you will find the clavipectoralis fascia, incise it, and retract medially the short head of the biceps and coracobrachialis. Do this with the arm adducted to protect the axillary artery and brachial plexus and retract the coracobrachialis carefully to protect the musculocutaneous nerve on its medial side. Beneath this muscles you will find the subscapularis covering the capsule; incise it, but use a stay suture to prevent it from disappearing medially. Then incise the capsule to reveal the humeral head.

If you are using a plate for the proximal humerus, be careful to put it lateral to the bicipital groove and the teres major tendon. Sometimes you will need to detach the pectoralis major tendon.

3. Dangers

Be careful with the musculocutaneous nerve in the coracobrachialis muscle; it lies 5 to 8 cm distal to the coracoid process.

The other structure you should be aware of is the cephalic vein. It should be preserved, but its ligation does not lead to big problems.

B. Lateral Approach to the Shoulder

1. Indications

- Open reduction and internal fixation (ORIF) of greater tuberosity fractures
- Intramedullary nailing of the humerus
- ORIF of humeral neck fractures

2. Position

- Supine or in beach chair
- Sandbag under the spine and the medial border of the scapula to push the shoulder forward and stabilize it

3. Incision

- Straight lateral 5-cm incision from the tip of the acromion to the lateral aspect of the deltoid

4. Surgical Dissection

Split the deltoid fibers for 5 cm and put a stay suture to prevent damage to the axillary nerve. Expose the rotator cuff and cut the coracoacromial ligament. Incise the rotator cuff in line with its fibers anterior to the acromion and adduct the arm to expose the proximal humerus and the tuberosities.

II. SURGICAL APPROACHES TO THE HUMERUS

A. Anterior Approach

1. Indications

- Proximal humeral fractures
- Middle-third shaft fractures

2. Position

Supine, with the arm in an arm board and abducted 60 degrees

3. Incision

Longitudinal from the tip of the coracoid to the deltopectoral groove straight to the deltoid insertion in the humerus and then following the lateral border of the biceps to 5 cm proximal to the flexion crease in the elbow (Fig. 1)

4. Surgical Dissection

The internervous plane is between the deltoid, axillary nerve, and the pectoralis major, medial, and lateral pectoral nerves proximally and the medial, musculo-cutaneous, lateral radial nerve, and fibers of the brachialis.

The proximal approach is the same as the deltopectoral or anterior approach to the shoulder. Distally, identify the interval between the biceps brachii and the brachialis and retract the biceps laterally to expose the brachialis (Figs. 2 and 3).

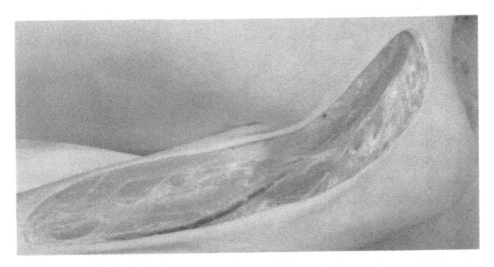

Figure 1   Anterior approach to the humerus: starts from the coracoid process to the deltopectoral groove and follows the lateral border of the biceps ending 5 cm proximal to the flexion crease of the elbow.

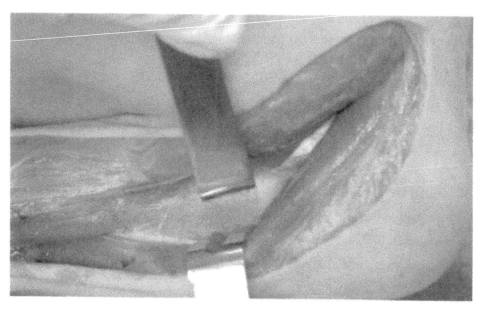

Figure 2 Anterior approach to the humerus: interval between the deltoid and biceps brachii muscles in the proximal humerus.

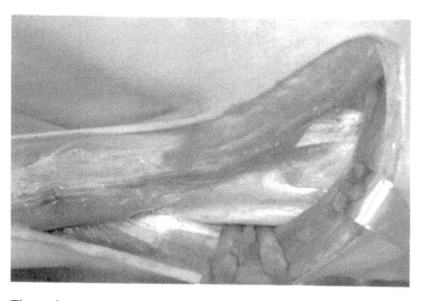

Figure 3 Anterior approach to the humerus: deep surgical dissection between the deltoid and biceps brachii muscles in the proximal humerus.

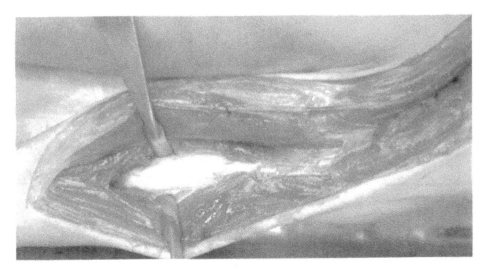

Figure 4 Anterior approach to the humerus: blunt dissection of the brachialis in the distal part of the humerus exposing the shaft.

Incise the periosteum of the humerus proximally, lateral to the pectoralis major insertion, if you need detach the pectoralis fro the lateral lip of the bicipital groove. Distally, dissect bluntly the brachialis in two halves to expose the shaft of the humerus (Fig. 4).

B. Anterolateral Approach

1. Indications

Fractures of the distal third of the humerus. It can be extended proximally and distally.

2. Position

Supine with the arm in an arm board and abducted 60 degrees

3. Incision

Curved lateral incision over the lateral border of the biceps following the muscle and ending at the flexion crease

4. Surgical Dissection

There is no true internervous plane and the radial nerve is at risk all the time.

Take care when dissecting in the fascia because the lateral cutaneous nerve of the forearm runs in line with the approach. Identify the biceps, retract it medially, expose the brachialis and brachioradialis, and identify the interval between these two muscles. Develop the interval between them (Figs. 5 and 6).

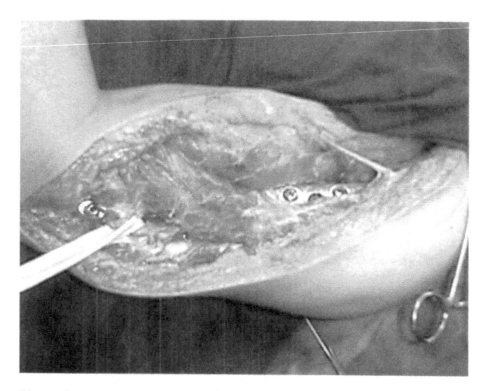

Figure 5   Anterolateral approach to the humerus: surgical exposure of a humeral shaft fracture, exposing the brachialis and brachioradialis.

Take care to find the radial nerve between the two muscles and trace it proximally to the lateral intermuscular septum; retract it laterally and incise the lateral border of the brachialis longitudinally to the bone. Elevate it subperiosteally medially to expose the humeral shaft.

C.   Posterior Approach

1.   Indications

All but upper 25% humeral shaft fractures—easily extensile to the elbow and forearm

2.   Position (Figs. 7 and 8)

- Prone and the arm in an arm board, arm abducted 60 degrees
- Lateral with the affected side up

3.   Incision (Fig. 9)

Starting 8 cm distal to the acromion and from there a straight longitudinal incision in the midline of the posterior aspect of the arm to the olecranon fossa.

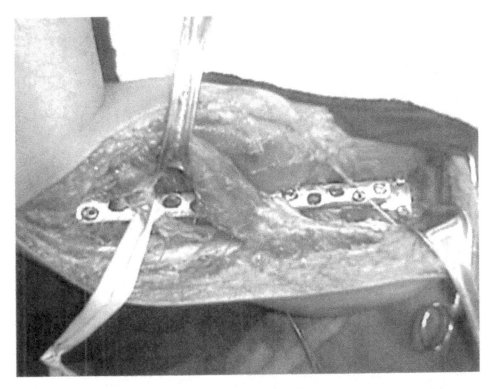

Figure 6   Anterolateral approach to the humerus: a Penrose drain holding the radial nerve. Observe the extended exposure of the humeral shaft from the head to the distal part.

4. Surgical Dissection

There is no internervous plane; dissection involves separating the lateral and long heads of the triceps, innervated by the radial nerve

Identify the gap between the long and the lateral heads. Begin proximally with blunt dissection and then incise the tendon distally. Retract the lateral head laterally and the long head medially (Figs. 10 and 11).

Then identify the radial nerve proximally to the insertion of the medial head of the triceps in the spiral groove. Put a Penrose drain around it to mark it during the procedure (Fig. 12).

Incise the medial head of the triceps by blunt dissection and strip the muscle subperiosteally to expose the humeral shaft (Figs. 13 and 14).

Gerwin, in a cadaver study, proposed a modified posterior approach, which extends the indications to 94% of the humeral shaft. The incision is the same, but first you have to retract the triceps medially, exposing the lateral brachial cutaneous nerve on the posterior aspect of the lateral intermusculaar septum and

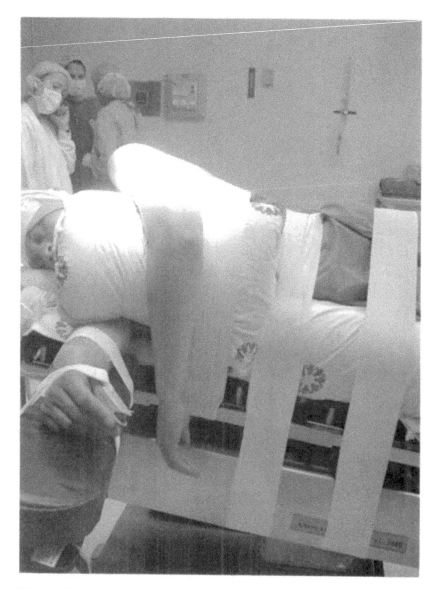

Figure 7 Posterior approach to the humerus: lateral decubitus position with a pillow under the arm.

trace it proximally and identify the main trunk of the radial nerve proximal to where it pierces the intermuscular septum. You then divide the septum distally for 3 cm to permit mobilization of the radial nerve. Elevate subperiosteally the medial and lateral heads medially and expose the humeral shaft. This approach can be extended to the axillary nerve.

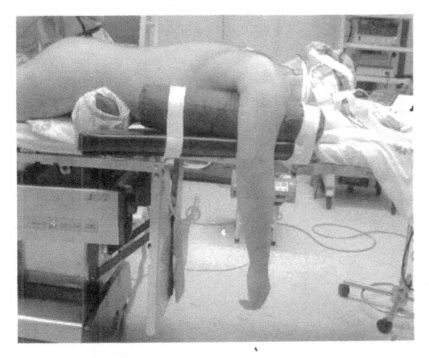

Figure 8   Posterior approach to the humerus: prone position.

D.   Medial Approach

1.   Indications

Obese patients with middle-third humeral shaft fractures distal to the pectoralis major

2.   Position

Supine with the arm in an arm board abducted 90 degrees and externally rotated

3.   Incision

Distal (5 cm) to the axilla in line with the brachial artery and the median nerve, crossing the antecubital fossa from medial to lateral

4.   Surgical Dissection

The internervous plane is between the brachialis, musculocutaneous nerve and triceps, and radial nerve. Mobilize the brachial artery, its venae, and the median nerve.

Elevate the biceps and brachialis from the anterior surface of the humeral shaft from the pectoralis to the coronoid fossa and expose the humeral shaft.

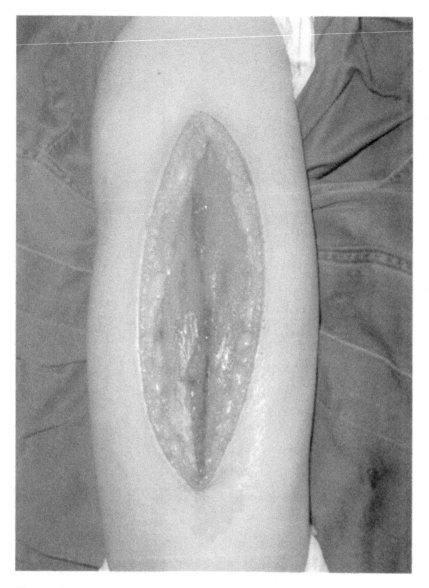

Figure 9   Posterior approach to the humerus: superficial incision—skin and subcutaneous tissue exposing the triceps muscle.

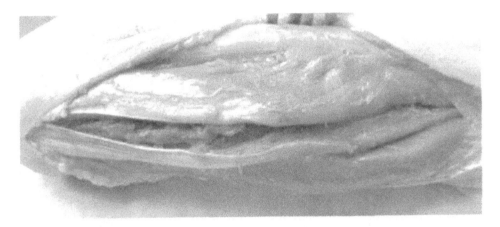

Figure 10   Posterior approach to the humerus: lateral and long heads of the triceps.

E. Lateral Approach

1. Indications

Distal humeral shaft fractures and fractures of the lateral condyle

2. Position

Supine with the arm across the chest

3. Incision

Straight incision over the lateral supracondylar ridge

4. Surgical Dissection

There is no internervous plane. The plane is between the triceps and the brachioradialis, both innervated by the radial nerve.

Incise the fascia in line with the skin. Identify the plane between the triceps and the brachioradialis and cut between them, retracting the brachioradialis anteriorly and the triceps posteriorly.

III. SURGICAL APPROACHES TO THE ELBOW

A. Anterior Approach

1. Indications

- Anterior capsular release
- Repair distal ruptures of the biceps tendon
- Graft the anterior neurovascular structures
- Resect heterotopic ossification

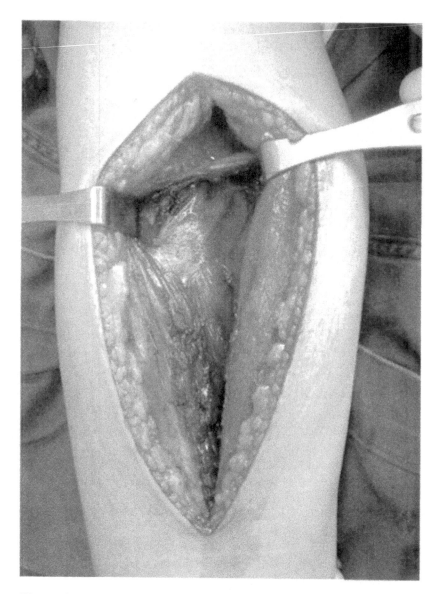

Figure 11 Posterior approach to the humerus: retract the lateral head laterally and the long head medially, exposing the radial nerve.

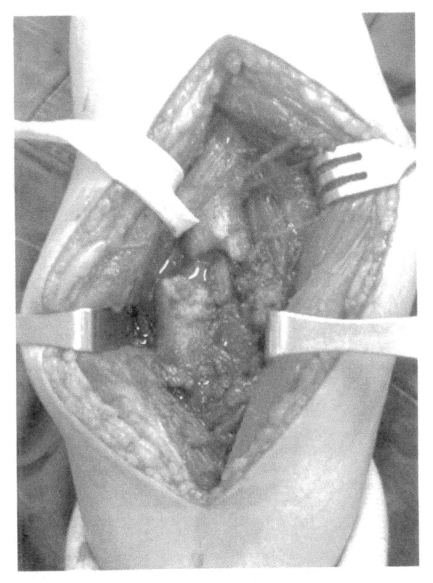

Figure 12 Posterior approach to the humerus: expose the radial nerve and put a Penrose drain around it to mark it throughout the procedure.

2. Position
    - Supine
    - Arm board
    - Tourniquet

3. Incision
    - Curved incision begins proximal and laterally at the medial side of the biceps.

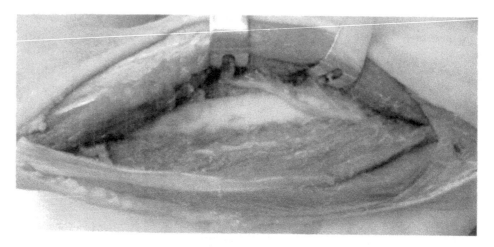

Figure 13 Posterior approach to the humerus: exposure of the humeral shaft and the radial nerve between the heads of the triceps.

- Incision crosses the elbow crease and proceeds toward the ulnar side of forearm; it extends distally following the medial border of the brachioradialis.

4. Surgical Dissection

The internervous plane is different proximally and distally. Proximally it is between the brachioradialis (radial) and brachialis (musculocutaneous) and distally between the brachioradialis (radial) and pronator teres (median).

Dissect the subcutaneous tissue and ligate the antecubital veins. Repair the lateral cutaneous nerve. Place a Penrose drain around the radial nerve and mobilize it laterally along with the common extensor origin.

Dissect distally to obtain capsular exposure. Preserve the medial antebrachial nerve medially.

Place a Penrose drain around the median nerve and brachial nerve and vein. Then identify the plane between the brachialis and the capsule. Place another Penrose drain around the brachialis to expose the capsule.

There are two possibilities for exposure of the capsule. If you retract the radial nerve and the common extensor origin laterally and the brachialis medially, you can expose the lateral half of the capsule, the anterior aspect of the proximal radioulnar joint, and the anterior aspect of the lateral collateral ligament complex. If you incise the capsule, you can expose the capitellum and the proximal radioulnar joint.

The second possible window is as follows: retract the brachialis laterally to expose the medial half of the capsule and the anterior part of the medial collateral ligament complex. If necessary, you can expose the coronoid fossa, but through a brachialis split.

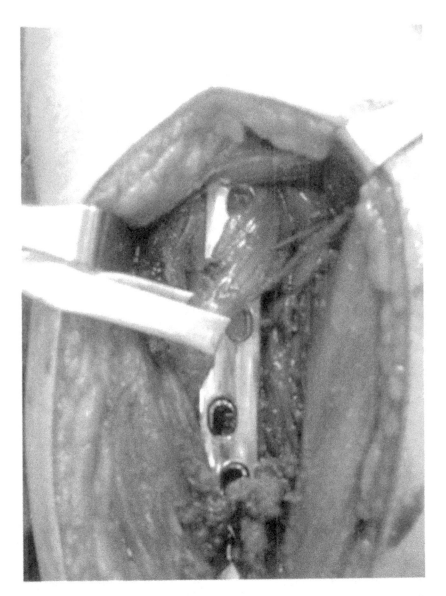

Figure 14   Posterior approach to the humerus: a DCP plate under the radial nerve.

5.   Dangers
   - The radial artery
   - The lateral cutaneous nerve of the forearm

B.   Posterior Approach

1.   Indications
   - Elbow arthroplasty
   - Fractures of the distal humerus

- Olecranon fractures
- Unreduced elbow dislocation
- Synovectomy
- Ankylosis

2. Position

- Prone decubitus
- Arm abducted 90 degrees
- Forearm flexed over the side of the table
- Tourniquet

3. Incision

A longitudinal incision begins above olecranon and just above the tip of the olecranon curve. The incision proceeds laterally and runs down to the lateral side of this curve. It is completed over the medial subcutaneous surface of the ulna.

3. Surgical Dissection

Identify the ulnar nerve in its groove and place a Penrose drain around it. Secure the drain with only a tight knot. Never use surgical clamps to secure it because traction will harm the nerve.

There are four basic choices for exposure the elbow joint:

- Triceps splitting. Described by Thompson in 1918, releasing the triceps from the ulna. Later on, the Van Gorder turndown was described by Campbell to allow increased flexion in severely contracted joints, but this required a long period of immobilization during its healing.
- Triceps reflecting. Preserve the triceps mechanism by reflecting it in continuity with the anconeus. We have two methods of doing this: (1) The Kocher posterolateral extensile triceps bearing enters the Kocher interval between the anconeus and the extensor carpi ulnaris. Elevate the anconeous with the triceps medially as a sleeve, preserving the distal attachment of the anconeous. (2) The Bryan Morrey technique reflects the triceps in continuity from medial to lateral, exposing and transposing the ulnar nerve. This same approach can be used with a flake of bone from the tip of the olecranon.
- Triceps preserving. Elevating and mobilizing the triceps both medially and laterally can expose the distal humerus.
- Olecranon osteotomy. There are many choices for this, but the most popular is V-type Chevron osteotomy. It is created at the midportion of the olecranon. The osteotomy is fixed with a screw or a tension band at the end of the procedure.

C. Lateral Approach

The lateral approach refers to the deep dissection, but you can use a posterior skin incision and dissect the subcutaneous tissue to expose the lateral part of the elbow. The position of the posterior interosseous nerve is important in performing any lateral approach to the elbow. Kaplan stressed the importance of performing this procedure with the forearm in pronation, which translates the nerve anteriorly, thus increasing the safe zone.

1. Indication

   - Radial head fractures
   - Capitellar fractures
   - Intraarticular fractures of the distal humerus
   - Lateral debridment of tennis elbow
   - Repair or reconstruction of the lateral collateral annular complex
   - Release of elbow contracture
   - Radial head resection or replacement

2. Position

   - Supine
   - Affected arm over the chest
   - Tourniquet

3. Incision

Begin over the posterior surface of the lateral humeral epicondyle and continue downward and medially to the posterior border of the ulna (Fig. 15).

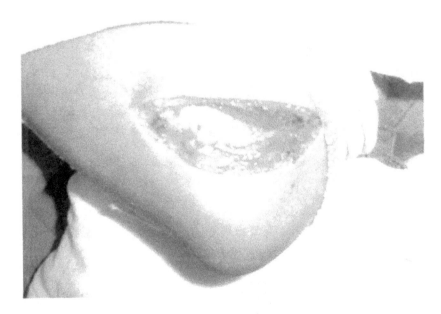

Figure 15 Lateral approach to the elbow: skin incision.

4. Surgical Dissection

There are different options:

- The direct lateral approach uses a direct longitudinal split through the lateral annular complex. A lateral incision starts from the lateral epicondyle and proceeds distally along the interval between anconeus and extensor carpi ulnaris. Then the lateral collateral ligament is incised in line with the forearm axis just anterior to the extensor carpi ulnaris to preserve the posterior fibers of the lateral collateral/annular complex. The incision can be extended for 4 cm distally before the posterior interosseous nerve is encountered.

- For the lateral-collateral–preserving approach, the incision follows the supracondylar ridge of the humerus and extends distally 3 cm posterior to the lateral epycondyle along the extensor carpi ulnaris and anconeus interval. The triceps and most proximal anconeus are reflected to expose the olecranon fossa and the posterolateral joint. Anterolateral joint exposure is obtained by dissecting of the brachioradialis and extensor carpis radialis longus from the lateral supracondylar ridge of the humerus. Exposure of the entire capsule is facilitated by dissection between the extensor carpi radialis longus and the extensor carpi radialis brevis. At the same time, the brachialis is elevated from the distal humerus and capsule, allowing exposure of the radial head.

- The lateral Kocher approach uses a single deep incision down the supracondylar ridge of the humerus and across the lateral epicondyle extended along the extensor carpi ulnaris and anconeus interval. The triceps and anconeous are reflected posteriorly with the posterior joint capsule and the common extensor origin, anterior capsule and lateral collateral ligament are reflected anteriorly (Figs. 16, 17, and 18). Enlargement of the approach requires the addition of a partial or complete detachment of the triceps tendon from its olecranon insertion.

- The anterolateral Kaplan approach lies between the extensor digitorum communis and the extensor carpi radialis longus. This interval is best found by observing where the vessels penetrate the anterior margin of the extensor digitorum communis aponeurosis. Split the fascia longitudinally and separate the extensor carpi radialis longus from the extensor digitorum communis . Deep to it lies the extensor carpi radialis brevis, and deep to this lies the supinator with the posterior interosseous nerve in its fibers surrounded by fat (Figs. 19 to 23) If you want to extend this approach, you should do it proximally, elevating the extensor carpi radialis longus, extensor carpi radialis brevis, and brachioradilais from the lateral supracondylar ridge of the humerus to expose the anterior joint capsule.

- The column procedure uses the Kaplan and Kocher approaches together. The extensor digitorum communis, the extensor carpi ulnaris, and the

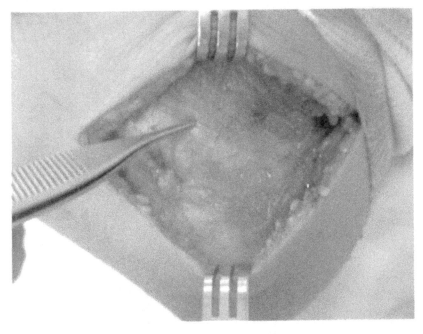

Figure 16 Lateral approach to the elbow—Kocher approach: superficial dissection showing the interval between the anconeous and the extensor carpi ulnaris.

lateral ulnar collateral ligament remain attached to the lateral epicondyle, preserving stability (Fig. 24).

D. Medial Approach

1. Indications

- Sinovectomy
- Removal of loose bodies
- Coronoid process fractures
- Medial humeral condylar and epicondylar fractures

2. Position

- Supine
- Arm board
- Abducted arm and externally rotated shoulder
- Tourniquet

3. Incision

Curved incision centering on the medial epicondyle.

4. Surgical Dissection

Palpate the ulnar nerve. Incise the fascia over the nerve, then isolate the nerve along the length of the incision.

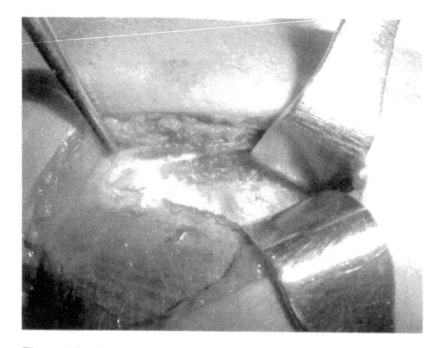

Figure 17 Lateral approach to the elbow—Kocher approach: superficial dissection showing the interval between the anconeous and the extensor carpi ulnaris exposing the joint capsule.

The superficial flexor muscles of the forearm are visible identified at the interval between the pronator teres and the brachialis muscles.

Retract the ulnar nerve inferiorly and perform an osteotomy of the medial epicondyle.

Incise the capsule and the medial collateral ligament and expose the joint.

5. Dangers

The ulnar nerve.

IV. SURGICAL APROACHES TO THE FOREARM

A. Anterior Approach

1. Indications

- ORIF of radial fractures
- Bone grafting
- Biopsy
- Radial osteotomy

2. Position

- Supine
- Arm board; forearm supination
- Tourniquet

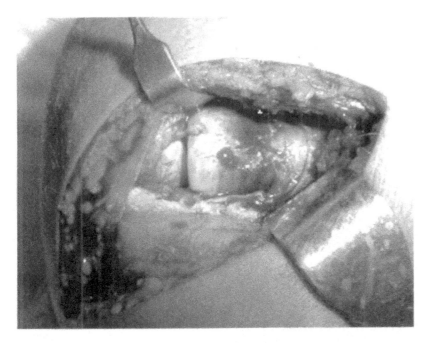

Figure 18   Lateral approach to the elbow—Kocher approach: superficial dissection showing the interval between the anconeous and the extensor carpi ulnaris exposing radial head.

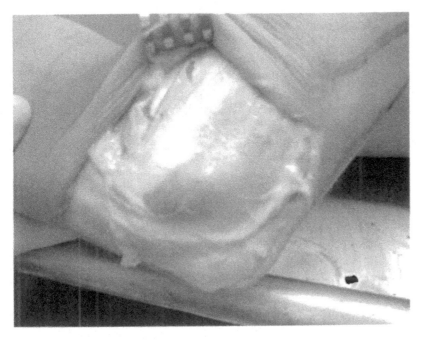

Figure 19   Lateral approach to the elbow—Anterolateral Kaplan apporach: skin incision.

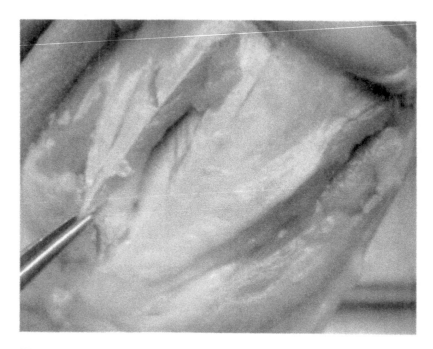

Figure 20   Lateral approach to the elbow—Anterolateral Kaplan approach: interval between the extensor carpi radialis longus and extensor digitorum communis.

3.   Incision

   • Straight incision between the elbow lateral to the biceps tendon down to the styloid process of the radius (Fig. 25).

4.   Surgical Dissection

   • Incise the skin and the fascia. Develop a plane between the flexor carpi radialis and the brachioradialis. Proximally, the plane is between the pronator teres and the brachioradialis.
   • Identify the superficial radial nerve underneath the brachioradialis. The radial artery lies beneath the brachioradialis. The artery may have to be mobilized medially (Fig. 26).

   Deep dissections are divided in thirds:

   • The proximal third is in relation to the biceps, following it to the insertion into the bicipital tuberosity. Incise the bursa to gain access to the radius proximally. The posterior interosseus nerve is located in relation to the supinator muscle. To avoid the nerve, displace it with fully supination laterally and posteriorly. According to Diliberti, there is a 3.8-cm safe zone distal to the radial head.
   • The middle-third is covered by the pronator teres and flexor digitorum

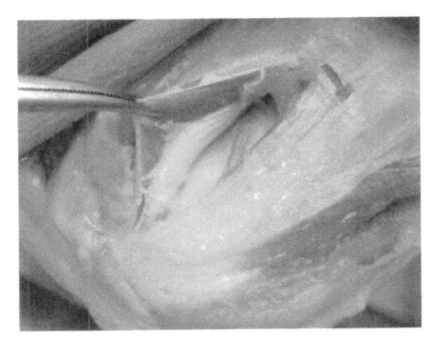

Figure 21   Lateral approach to the elbow—Anterolateral Kaplan approach: interval between the extensor carpi radialis longus and extensor digitorum communis, exposing the extensor carpi radialis brevis.

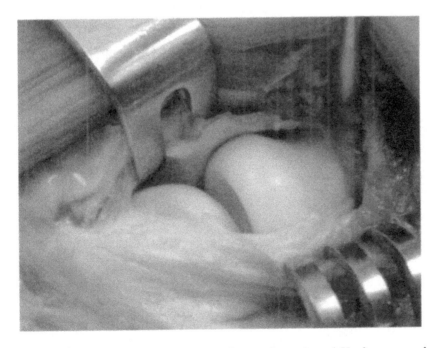

Figure 22   Lateral approach to the elbow—Anterolateral Kaplan approach: capsulotomy exposing the radial head and capitellum.

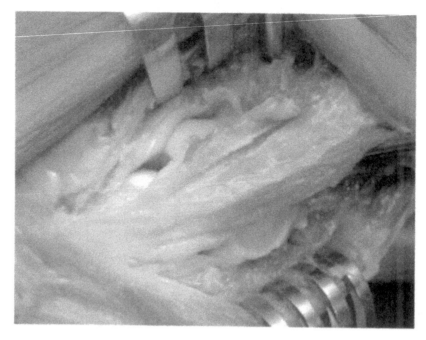

Figure 23 Lateral approach to the elbow—Column procedure: Extensor Digitorum Communis, Extensor Carpi Ulnaris and lateral collateral ulnar ligament remain attached to the lateral epicondyle.

superficialis. Pronate the forearm to expose the pronator teres insertion, detach this insertion, and strip the muscle to gain access to the bone.
- Distal third. first supinate the forearm and incise the periosteum lateral to the pronator quadratus and the flexor pollicis longus to gain access to the bone (Fig. 27).

5. Dangers

- The posterior interosseous nerve.
- The superficial radial nerve.
- The radial artery.

B. Approach via the Shaft of the Ulna

1. Indications

- ORIF of ulnar fractures
- Delayed union and nonunions of the ulna
- Osteotomy of the ulna
- Ulnar lengthening
- Osteomyelitis of the ulna

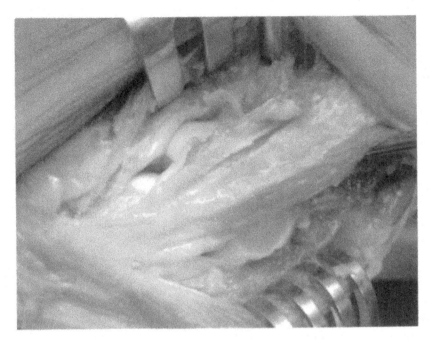

Figure 24 Lateral approach to the elbow—Column procedure combination of Kaplan and Kocher approaches: Extensor Digitorum Communis, Extensor Carpi Ulnaris and lateral collateral ulnar ligament remain attached to the lateral epicondyle.

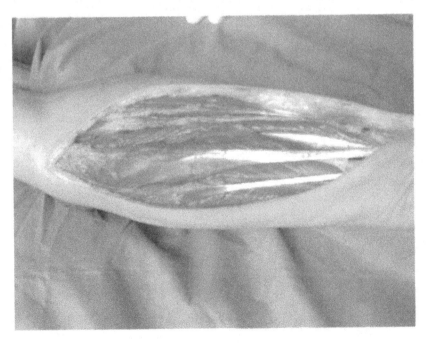

Figure 25 Anterior approach to the forearm: longitudinal incision from the elbow lateral to the biceps tendon down to the styloid process of the radius.

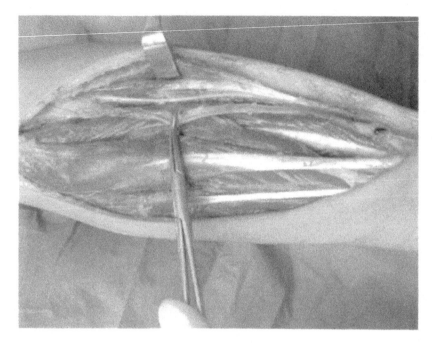

Figure 26 Anterior approach to the forearm: superficial radial nerve underneath the brachioradialis.

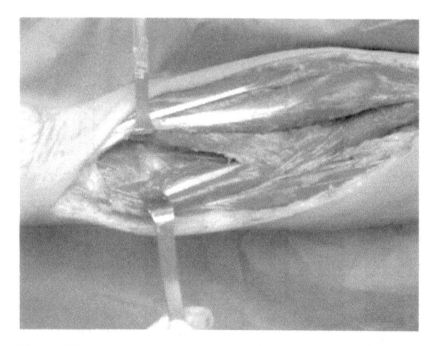

Figure 27 Anterior approach to the forearm distal third: exposure of the pronator quadratus.

2. Position

    - Supine
    - Arm across the chest
    - Tourniquet

3. Incision

    - Longitudinal over the subcutaneous border of the ulna

4. Surgical Dissection

    - Incision of the skin and fascia
    - Incision between the extensor carpi ulnaris and flexor carpi ulnaris exposing the shaft of the ulna

5. Dangers

    - Ulnar nerve
    - Ulnar artery

C. **Posterior Approach**

1. Indications

    - ORIF of radial fractures
    - Treatment of nonunions and delayed union
    - Decompression of the interosseous nerve
    - Radial osteotomy
    - Biopsy

2. Position

    - Supine
    - Arm board
    - Supination of the forearm
    - Tourniquet

3. Indication

    - Straight incision from a point anterolateral to the lateral epicondyle to the ulnar side of the Lister's tubercle

4. Surgical Dissection

    - Incise the skin and the fascia. Identify the interval between the extensor carpi brevis and the extensor digitorum communis. Identify the next plane between the extensor carpi radialis brevis and extensor digitorum communis. Continue the dissection to separate the two muscles and identify the shaft.
    - The supinator is located on the proximal third, and the posterior interosseus nerve runs with it. This approach is risky for this third.
    - Middle third the plane is between the adductor pollicis longus and the extensor pollicis brevis.

- Distal third of the plane is between the extensor carpi radialis brevis and the extensor pollicis longus.

5. Dangers

Posterior interosseous nerve

V. CONCLUSION

We have reviewed the different options to approach the upper extremity. As indicated throughout the chapter, there is a complex anatomy that must be taken care of in order to perform a safe and successful procedure. Sometimes, in difficult situations, the approaches may have to be combined.

Learning the anatomy and the surgical approaches are the first steps and the keys to optimal preoperative planning and to achieving the best possible results.

BIBLIOGRAPHY

1. S Hoppenfield P DeBoer. Surgical Exposures in Orthopaedics: The Anatomic Approach, Philadelphia: Lippincott, 1984, pp 1–139.
2. S D Patterson, GI Bain, JA Metha. Surgical approaches to the elbow. Clin Orthop 370:19–33, 2000.
3. EB Kaplan. Surgical approach to the proximal end of the radius and its use in fractures of the head and neck of the radius. J Bone Joint Surg 23:86–92,1941.
4. JM Wilkinson D Stanley. Posterior surgical approaches to the elbow: a comparative anatomic study. J Shoulder Elbow Surg 2001; 10(4):380–382.
5. M Gerwin, RN Hotchkiss, AJ Weiland. Alternative operative exposures of the posterior aspect of the humeral diaphysis with reference to the radial nerve. J Bone Joint Surg Am 1996;78(11):1690–1695.
6. BF Morrey. General deep approaches to the elbow: Posterior exposures. Techn Shoulder Elbow Surg 3(1):6–9, 2002.
7. RR Richards. General deep approaches: Anterior approaches. Techn Shoulder Elbow Surg 3(1):16–22, 2002.
8. H Hastings M Cohen. General deep approaches: Lateral approaches. Techn Shoulder Elbow Surg 3(1):10–15, 2002.
9. S Kozin, B Hines. Anatomical approach to the pronator teres. Techniques in hand and upper extremity surgery. Tech Hand Upper Extrem Surg 6(3): 152–154, 2002.
10. BF Morrey. Bryan-Morrey triceps-reflecting approach. Techn Shoulder Elbow Surg 3(1):28–32, 2002
11. D Ring J Jupiter. Surgical exposure to coronoid fractures. Techn Shoulder Elbow Surg 3(1):48–56, 2002.
12. CS Barlett. Elbow Fractures, Curr Opin Orthop 11:290–304, 2000.
13. G Marra M Stover. Glenoid and scapular body fractures. Curr Opin Orthop 10: 283–288, 1999.
14. G Gramstad G Marra. Treatment of genoid factures. Techn Shoulder Elbow Surg 3(2):102–110, 2002.

15. MT Mazurek AY Shin. Upper extremity peripheral nerve anatomy, current concepts and applications. Clin Orthop 383:7–20, 2001.

16. G King. Surgical Exposure for open reduction and internal fixation or prosthetic replacement of the radial head. Techn Shoulder Elbow Surg 3(1):39–47, 2002.

17. DC Dykes, RF Kyle, AH Schmidt. Operative treatment of humeral shaft Fractures: Plates vs nails. Techni Shoulder Elbow Surg 2(3):194–209, 2001.

18. JM Wilkinson D Stanley. Posterior surgical approaches to the elbow: A comparative anatomic study. J Shoulder Elbow Surg 10(4):380–382, 2001.

19. GJW King. Superficial Surgical Exposures of the Elbow. Techn Shoulder Elbow Surg 3(1):2–5, 2002.

20. SW O'Driscoll. Triceps-anconeous pedicle approach for distal humerus fractures and nonunions. Techni in Shoulder Elbow Surg 3(1):33–38, 2002.

21. MA Frankle. Triceps Split technique for total elbow arthroplasty. Techn Shoulder Elbow Surg 3(1):23–27, 2002.

22. PA Dowdy, GI Bain, GJW King, SD Patterson. The midline posterior elbow incision, an anatomical appraisal. J Bone Joint Surg 77-B:696–699, 1995.

23. SW O'Driscoll, E Horii, SW Carmichael, B Morrey. The cubital tunnel and ulnar neuropathy. J Bone Joint Surg 73-B:613–617, 1991.

24. JB Jupiter. Complex non-union of the humeral diaphysis. Treatment with a medial approach, an anterior plate, and a vascularized fibular graft. J Bone Joint Surg 72-A:701–707, 1990.

25. M Spinner. The arcade of Frohse and its relationship to posterior interossoues nerve paralysis. J Bone Joint Surg 50-B:809–812, 1968.

26. RO Whitson. Relation of the radial nerve to the shaft of the humerus. J Bone Joint Surg 36-A:85–88, 1954.

27. P Mansat, BF Morrey. The column procedure: A limited lateral approach for extrinsic contracture of the elbow. J Bone Joint Surg 80-A:1603–1615, 1998.

28. RS Bryan, BF Morrey. Extensive posterior exposure of the elbow. A triceps sparing approach. Clin Orthop 166:188–192, 1982.

29. WJ Mills, DP Hanel, DG Smith. Lateral approach to the humeral shaft: An alternative for fracture treatment. J Orthop Trauma 10(2):81–86, 1996.

30. RL Uhl, JM Larosa, T Sibeni, LJ Martino. Posterior approaches to the humerus: When should you worry about the radial nerve? J Orthop Trauma 10(5):338–340, 1996.

31. T Diliberti, MJ Botte, RA Abrams. Anatomical considerations regarding the posterior interosseous nerve during posterolateral approaches to the proximal part of the radius. J Bone Joint Surg 82A (6):809–813, 2000.

Index